耳から学ぶ
楽しいナース英語

中西睦子／監修
野口ジュディー・川越栄子・仁平雅子／著

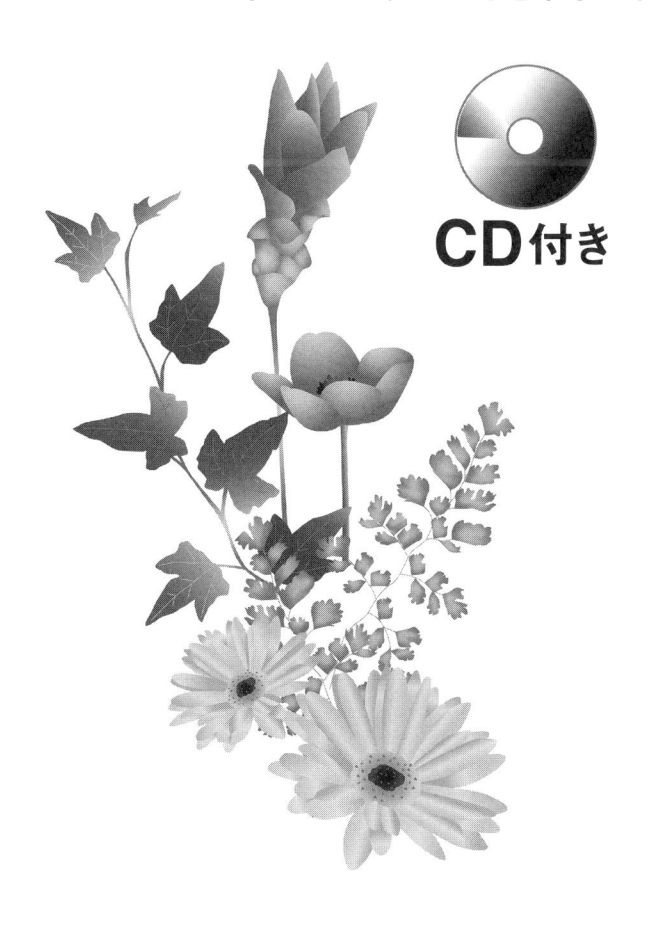

CD付き

講談社サイエンティフィク

はじめに

　「国際化」「グローバル化」が叫ばれている今日，海外から多くの人々が日本を訪れ，仕事をされたり，学んだりしておられます．そのおり，体調を崩して病院を訪れる外国人患者さんも年々増えてきています．患者さんの国籍は様々でしょうが，ナースも世界共通語とされる英語でケアをする機会が今後ますます増えていくでしょう．その際，最低限必要なコミュニケーションを英語で行う能力が必要とされます．

　英語でコミュニケーションをするというと，日本人はとても難しいように感じる人が多いかもしれません．しかし，病院のケアの場面で使う英語は，中学校で習った基本単語と少しの専門用語を学ぶだけで充分通じるのです．英語が苦手だと考えている人も本書で学んでいただければ，「なんだ，こんなに簡単だったのか」ときっと驚かれると思います．そのためには，まず「耳から学ぶ」ことが第一です．

　本書では，この「耳から学ぶ」という，外国語習熟のために一番重要なところを始めるための入門書です．本書は14のユニットで構成されていますが，それぞれのユニットは，入院および外来でのケア場面ごとに作られています．

　まずTalkで基本的な会話を紹介します．次にLessonで必ず覚えておきたい用語，表現をあげてあります．このTalkとLessonをCDで繰り返し聴いてください．「繰り返し聴く」ことがポイントです．通学・通勤途上の電車の中でも，職場・学校，どこでも，少し時間があったら，音楽CDで聴くように何度も何度も聴いてください．そうしていると，不思議なことに英語のフレーズが自然に頭に入ってしまいます．そして，何も考えないでも口から出てくるようになります．これは，私たちが幼いとき，耳から日本語を聞いていて，意識せずに話せるようになったのと同じプロセスです．

　次にExerciseに挑戦してみてください．TalkとLessonを何度も聴いた人には決して難しくはありません．それに続いて「知っておきたい用語」「応用フレーズ」へと学習を広げてください．これらはCDには録音されていませんが，きっとあなたの表現を豊かにしてくれます．

　なお，英語の表現に関して，また異なった文化を持っておられる患者さんへの対応について，現場のナースの苦労話なども交えたコラムをのせました．参考にしてください．

　本書は，「耳から」「楽しんで」学んでいただくものです．ミュージックを楽しむように

気楽に，マイペースでどうぞ．この一冊をマスターすれば，外国人患者さんが来られても，日常のケアにはあまり困らないはずです．英語でコミュニケーションできる頼もしいナースになってください．

Please enjoy yourself！

2002年3月

中　西　睦　子

目　　次　Contents

Unit 1	**I'm your primary nurse.** 私があなたのプライマリーナースです
Unit 2	**I'd like to ask you some questions.** あなたのことをきかせてください
Unit 3	**What is worrying you the most?** あなたの気がかりは何でしょうか
Unit 4	**Let me show you around the ward.** 病棟をご案内します
Unit 5	**Let's make a care plan.** ケアプランを立てましょう
Unit 6	**What is 'informed consent'?** 「インフォームドコンセント」って何ですか
Unit 7	**What kind of pain is it?** どのように痛みますか
Unit 8	**We'll do some tests.** 検査をしましょう
Unit 9	**Let's start your treatment.** 処置をしましょう
Unit 10	**Please take this medicine.** 薬を飲んでください
Unit 11	**I'm sure the results will be good.** きっといい結果になりますよ
Unit 12	**Now, you can leave the hospital.** いよいよ退院ですね
Unit 13	**In the outpatient department** 病院外来で
Unit 14	**At the clinic** 診療所で
Appendix	**Children's world, children's words** 子供の世界，子供のことば

Unit 1 — I'm your primary nurse.
私があなたのプライマリーナースです

Talk 1

Ns : Hello, Mr. Smith.　I'm Junko Ito.
　　（こんにちは，スミスさんですね．伊藤純子です）

Pt : Hello, Ms. Ito.
　　（こんにちは，伊藤さん）

Ns : I'm your primary nurse.　Please feel free to ask me anything.
　　（私がプライマリーナースです．何でもお聞きになってくださいね）

Pt : That will be of great help to me.　I cannot speak Japanese very well.
　　（助かります．私は日本語があまりできません）

Ns : I can speak English a little.　Please speak slowly.
　　（私は英語を少し話せます．ゆっくり話してくださいね）

◆ **'Please feel free to ask me anything.'**（何でもおききになってくださいね）◆

入院した患者さんは通常は口にしなくてもいいこと，時には恥ずかしいこともナースに，たずねたり，話さなければならない場合があります．その気持ちを和らげていただくのに大変役に立つ表現です．

次のフレーズも覚えておくと便利な表現です．

'Please do not hesitate to ask me anything.'
　　　　　（ためらわないで（遠慮なく），気軽にたずねてください）

'Please don't be shy'　　　　　（恥ずかしがらないでください）

Lesson 1

①入ってもいいですか	May I come in?
②おはようございます ～さん	Good morning, Mr. ～
③こんにちは ～さん	Good afternoon, Mr. ～
④こんばんは ～さん	Good evening, Ms. ～
⑤すみません，失礼します（その場を離れる時）	Excuse me. I have to go now.
⑥すぐに戻ってきます	I'll come back soon.
⑦またあとで	See you later.

⑧どうぞこちらへ	This way please.
⑨ここがあなたのお部屋，567号室です	Here is your room, Room 567.
⑩この部屋は4人部屋です	This room is for four people.
⑪同室の方をご紹介します	Let me introduce you to your roommates.
⑫この部屋は個室です	This room is a private room.
⑬こちらがあなたのベッドです	This is your bed.

⑭持ち物はロッカーに入れてください	Please put your belongings in the locker.
⑮貴重品はロッカーに入れないでください	Please do not keep valuables in the locker.
⑯貴重品は病室におかないでください	Please do not leave valuables in the hospital room.
⑰タオルはこの引出しに入れてください	Please put your towels in the drawer.
⑱こちらが寝衣です	Here is your hospital gown.

⑲朝食は8時，昼食は12時，夕食は5時です

　　　　Breakfast is served at 8, lunch at noon, and supper at 5.

⑳（食事の）トレイはワゴンにお返しください

　　　　Please return the tray to the wagon.

㉑男性は月，水，金に入浴できます

　　　　Men can take baths on Mondays, Wednesdays, and Fridays.

㉒女性は火，木，土に入浴できます

　　　　Women can take baths on Tuesdays, Thursdays, and Saturdays.

㉓入浴は午前8時～午後8時までいつでもできます

　　　　You can take a bath anytime from 8:00 a.m. to 8:00 p.m.

㉔面会時間は月曜から金曜までは午後3時から7時までです
　　　　　　　　　　　　　　　　Visiting hours are from 3:00 p.m. to 7:00 p.m. on weekdays.
㉕消灯時間は午後9時です　　　　　Lights-out is 9:00 p.m.
㉖電気を消してください　　　　　　Please turn off the light.
㉗あちらの公衆電話が使えます　　　You can use the pay phone over there.
㉘ここで携帯電話は使ってはいけません　You cannot use cellular phones here.
㉙この案内書を読んでください　　　Please read this guide.
㉚ナースコールのテストをしましょう　Let's try out the call button.
㉛ナースをよぶときにはこのボタンをこのように押してください
　　　　　　　　　　　　　　　　Push this button like this to call the nurse.
㉜何か質問はありませんか　　　　　Do you have any questions?

『あいさつは会話の始まり』

　その日初めて患者さんに会うときは，午前中ならば 'Good morning'，午後は 'Good afternoon'，夕食以降は 'Good evening' と必ず言い，その後患者さんのお名前を呼んでください．

　'Good morning, Mr. Smith' というように先ず声をかけてから用件に入ってください．患者さんはご自分のお名前を呼ばれることで，とてもナースに親近感，信頼感，安心感をもたれます．ケアをする上で大変重要なことです．様々な場面で出来る限りお名前を呼ぶように心がけましょう．

　また少しくだけた言い方で 'Hello'（おはよう/こんにちは/こんばんは）を使ってもいいです．これは，一日中使える表現です．

Exercise 1

Listen to the CD and fill in the blanks.
（CDを聞いて，下線部分をうめなさい）

1. _____ _____ are from 2:00 p.m. to 8:00 p.m.
   （面会時間は午後2時から8時までです）
2. You can _____ ___ _____ every day.
   （毎日入浴できます）
3. Please try to sleep after _____.
   （消灯時間以降は眠るように努力してください）
4. You can _____ _____ _____ at home tomorrow.
   （明日外泊しても結構です）
5. I'll _____ _____ in an hour.
   （1時間以内にまた来ます）
6. Please read this _____.
   （このパンフレットを読んでください）
7. Can I keep some coins in the _____?
   （小銭は引き出しに入れていいですか）
8. May I push the _____ _____ like this?
   （ナースコールはこのように押していいのですか）
9. Where should I keep my _____?
   （貴重品はどこにおいておけばよいのでしょうか）
10. Can I use the _____ _____ with a telephone card?
    （公衆電話はテレフォンカードが使えますか）

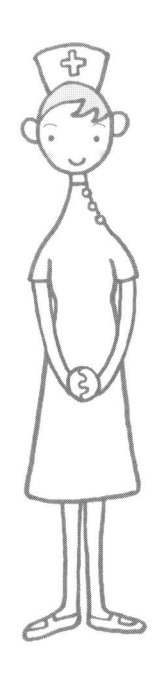

知っておきたい用語

入院患者	ínpatient	回診	rounds
入院	hospitalizátion	起床時間	wáke-up time
	admíssion	食事時間	méaltime
入院する	be in hóspital,	消灯時間	bédtime
	be hóspitalized		líghts-óut
退院する	be dischárged,	面会者，見舞い客	vísitor
	leave the hóspital	「面会謝絶」	No vísitors
外出する	go out	洗面用具	daily care ítems
外泊する	stay out óvernight	入れ歯	false teeth
病院の金庫	hóspital safe	小銭	change, coin
パンフレット	brochure [brouʃur]	上履き	slíppers

「プライマリーナース」

　病院にもよりますが，入院患者さんお一人ずつに担当のナースがつくことが増えてきました．これはプライマリーナーシングの考え方によるものです．

　'Primary nurse' という名称は，その発祥の地，アメリカのミネソタ大学のM.Mantheyさんが言い始めた言葉です．このprimary nurse（第一の/主な　ナース）には2つの意味があります．

　すなわち患者さんのケアを「第一に，主に」行うナースという意味と，もう1つは，患者さんと「1対1」の関係にあるナースという意味です．

　ナースの仕事は効率よくチームで分担されていますが，それだけでは患者さんから見て，誰が自分の看護に責任を持ってくれるのかわかりにくいでしょう．「おーい，誰に相談したらいいんだい？」というときに，看護チームのいわば「顔」になるのがこのプライマリーナースです．

　プライマリーナースの名称には，二人の人間が向き合うところから始まる，看護の仕事の原型が隠されていたのですね．

************** 応用フレーズ **************

担当ナースは8時間ごとに交替します　　The nurses are on 8-hour shifts.
ナースは午後4時，深夜12時と午前8時に交替します
　　　　　　　　　　　The nurses change shifts at 4:00 p.m., 12:00 p.m. and 8:00 a.m.
現金はご家族の方に家に持って帰ってもらってください
　　　　　　　　　　　　　　　Please ask your family to take any cash home.
面会時間は土曜，日曜，祝日は午前10時から午後7時までです．
　　　　Visiting hours are from 10:00 a.m. to 7:00 p.m. on Saturdays, Sundays and holidays.
面会は30分以内に制限されています　　You can visit the patient only for 30 minutes.
一度に3人を越えての入室はご遠慮ください
　　　　　　　　　　　　　　Only up to three people can enter the room at one time.
電気器具の使用は使用許可を得てください
　　　　　　　　　　　　Please request permission before using electrical appliances.
セルフサービスのコインランドリーと，ランドリーサービスがご利用いただけます．
　　　　　　　　　　　　We have a self-service coin laundry and a laundry service.
院外へ出るときはナースにお知らせください
　　　　　　　　　　　Please let us know, if you wish to temporarily leave the hospital.
喫煙所でしか煙草はすえません　　You can smoke only in designated smoking areas.
喫煙所は面会室に設けています　　The smoking area is in the patients' lounge.
1階ロビーに国際通話できる電話があります
　　　　　　　We have a pay phone for international calls.　It's in the lobby on the first floor.

◆　'Please speak slowly.'（ゆっくり話してくださいね）◆
　母国語が英語の方に普通のスピードで英語を話されると大変聴き取りにくいものです．日本人の中には充分理解できていないのに，わかったふりをしてしまう人もいるようです．しかし，ケアの現場で，そのようなことをすると大きな事故にもつながることになります．恥ずかしがらずに，本当にわかるまで聞き返しましょう．相手の言っていることがわからない時は次の表現で聞きましょう．
　　I beg your pardon? /　Pardon（me）? / Please say that again.
　　　　　　　　　　　　　　（もう一度言っていただけませんか）
　　Please speak more slowly.　　　（もう少しゆっくり言っていただけませんか）

Unit 2 — I'd like to ask you some questions.
あなたのことをきかせてください

Talk 2

Ns : I'd like to ask you some questions.
　　（あなたのことをきかせてください）

Pt : OK
　　（わかりました）

Ns : Are you living in Japan alone?
　　（日本にお一人で住んでおられますか）

Pt : Yes.　I've been living in Japan for 6 months on business.
　　My family is living in the U.S.
　　（はい．仕事で今までで6ヶ月日本にいます．家族はアメリカにいます）

Ns : Whom should we contact in an emergency?
　　（緊急の際はどなたに連絡すればよいですか）

Pt : Please contact Mr. Yamada.　He's one of my friends.　His telephone number is 331-2967.
　　（友人の山田さんにお願いします．電話番号は331-2967です）

Ns : Now I have some questions about your health condition.
　　（次に健康状態について質問させてください）

Pt : OK
　　（わかりました）

Ns : How is your appetite?
　　（食欲はありますか）

Pt : I've had no appetite recently.　I eat only once or twice a day.
　　（いいえ．最近食欲がなくて，1日に1回か2回です）

Ns : Is there anything else that's bothering you?
　　（他に具合の悪いところはありませんか）

Pt : I have a slight headache.
　　（少々頭痛がします）

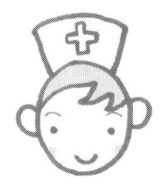

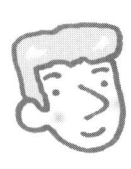

Lesson 2

Nurse

① どちらから来られたのですか　　Where are you from?
② 以前に大きな病気をしたことがありますか
　　　　　　　　　　　　　　　　Have you ever had a serious illness before?
③ 入院したことがありますか　　　Have you ever been hospitalized?
④ 食欲はどうですか　　　　　　　How is your appetite?
　　　　　　　　　　　　　　　　Do you have an appetite?
⑤ 間食はされていましたか　　　　Do you eat snacks between meals?
⑥ よく眠れますか　　　　　　　　Can you sleep well?
⑦ 昼寝をされていましたか　　　　Do you take naps during the day?

⑧ 煙草を吸いますか　　　　　　　Do you smoke?
⑨ 1日にどのくらい煙草を吸いますか　How many cigarettes do you smoke per day?
⑩ お酒は飲みますか　　　　　　　Do you drink alcohol?
⑪ 1日にどのくらいお酒を飲みますか　How much alcohol do you drink in a day?
⑫ アレルギーはありますか　　　　Are you allergic to anything?

⑬ 薬に対するアレルギーはありますか　Are you allergic to any medications?
⑭ 食物に対するアレルギーはありますか　Are you allergic to any food?
⑮ 毎日正常な便通がありますか　　Do you have regular and normal bowel movements?
⑯ 尿は1日何回ぐらいしますか　　How many times do you urinate per day?
⑰ 生理は順調ですか　　　　　　　Are your periods regular?
⑱ 何か常用している薬はありますか　Are you taking any medication regularly?
⑲ ご家族に同じ病気の方はおられますか
　　　　　　　　　　　　　　　　Is there anyone in your family who has the same illness?
⑳ 宗教上食べられないものはありますか
　　　　　　　　　　　　　　　　Is there anything you cannot eat for a religious reason?

Patient

㉑ 食欲がありません　　　　　　　I have no appetite.
㉒ 食欲がほとんどありません　　　I have little appetite.

㉓常に疲れた感じがします	I always feel tired.	(I feel exhausted.)
㉔力が抜けたような感じがします	I feel weak.	(I feel lethargic.)
㉕めまいがします	I feel dizzy.	
㉖いらいらします	I feel irritated.	
㉗眠れません	I can't sleep.	(I'm suffering from insomnia.)
㉘左手がしびれます	My left hand feels numb.	
㉙体重が減っています	I'm losing weight.	
㉚頭痛がします	I have a headache.	
㉛肩がこります	I have stiff shoulders.	
㉜腰が痛いです	I have a backache.	
㉝汗をかいています	I'm sweating.	
㉞熱があります	I have a fever.	
㉟熱が高いです	I have a high fever.	
㊱熱が少しあります	I have a slight fever.	
㊲体が熱っぽいです	I feel feverish.	
㊳寒気がします	I feel chilly.	
㊴ぞくぞくします	I feel shaky.	
㊵胃（お腹）が痛いです	I have a stomachache.	
㊶吐き気がします	I feel nauseated.	
㊷むかむかします	I feel like vomiting.	
㊸下痢をしています	I have diarrhea.	(I have loose bowels)
㊹便秘をしています	I'm constipated.	(便秘 : constipation)
㊺げっぷがでます	I burp a lot.	
㊻しゃっくりがとまりません	I can't stop hiccuping.	
㊼吐血しました	I vomited blood.	
㊽尿がでにくいです	I have difficulty urinating.	
㊾トイレが近いです	I need to urinate very often.	
㊿失禁します	I'm incontinent.	
(51)血尿がでます	I have bloody urine.	

(52)声がかすれます	I have a hoarse voice.
(53)咳がとまりません	I can't stop coughing.
(54)よくくしゃみがでます	I sneeze a lot.
(55)のどが痛いです	I have a sore throat.
(56)鼻血がでます	I have a nose bleed.
(57)耳鳴りがします	I have a ringing in my ears.
(58)よく聞こえないのです	I have difficulty hearing.

(59)貧血気味です	I'm anemic.
(60)貧血で倒れました	I collapsed from anemia.
(61)動悸が激しいです	I'm suffering from palpitations.
(62)不整脈があります	I have an irregular pulse.
(63)息苦しいです	I have difficulty breathing.
(64)息切れがします	I get short of breath.

(65)かゆいです	I feel itchy.
(66)体中がかゆいです	My body itches all over.
(67)発疹がでています	I have a skin eruption.
(68)目が痛いです	My eyes hurt.
(69)目がかゆいです	My eyes feel itchy.
(70)目がかすみます	I have bleary eyes.

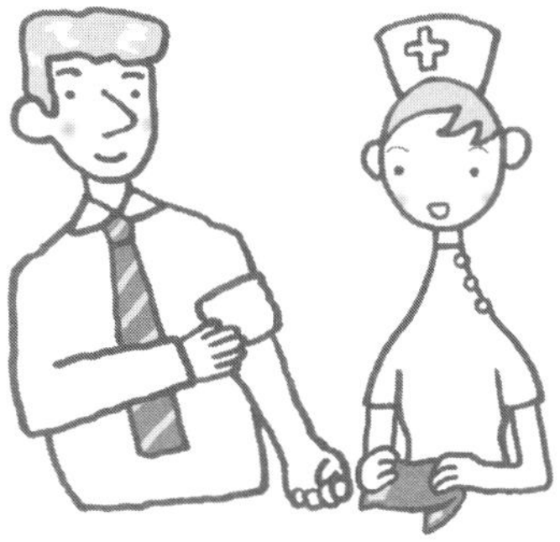

Exercise 2

Listen to the CD and fill in the blanks.
(CDを聞いて，下線部分をうめなさい)

1. What seems to be the greatest _____?
   （一番の問題は何ですか）
2. How many _____ do you _____ every day?
   （毎日睡眠は何時間とっていますか）
3. What food are you _____ to?
   （どんな食物に対してアレルギーがありますか）
4. Do you feel _____?
   （目まいはしますか）
5. Do you often have _____?
   （しばしば下痢をしますか）
6. I am sometimes _____.
   （時々便秘をします）
7. I collapsed from _____ a week ago.
   （1週間前貧血で倒れました）
8. I drink alcoholic bevarages _____ _____ a week.
   （1週間に3回お酒をのみます）
9. I always feel _____.
   （いつもいらいらしています）
10. My stomach _____ _____ after I eat.
    （食べた後胃がもたれます）

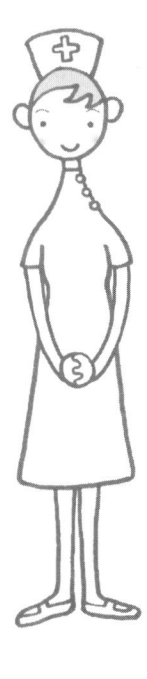

知っておきたい用語

他覚症状

咳	cough	切り傷	cut
痰	spútum	噛み傷	bite
眼の充血	blood shot of eyes	刺し傷	sting
黄疸	jáundice	引っかき傷	scratch
浮腫	edéma	打撲傷	bruise
発疹	rash	傷あと	scar
湿疹	éczema	かさぶた	crust
水疱	blíster	床ずれ	bédsore
腫脹	swélling	しもやけ	fróstbite
しこり	lump	にきび	pímples
こぶ	bump	じんましん	híves
心雑音	heart múrmur	光過敏	light sensitívity
硬直	rigídity	瞳孔散大	dilátion of the pupil
昏睡状態	coma	血便（尿）	bloody stool（urine）

『どこからがプライバシー？』

「ここからが私のプライバシー」と感じる一線は，人によってずいぶん違うようです．

アメリカで，指導教授のお宅に招かれたある日本人学生は，訪問先の応接間でくつろいでいた男性を「彼，私の別れた夫よ」と紹介されてびっくりしたそうです．その学生は，指導教授の「隠された過去」にまで踏み込むつもりはまったくなかったので，これは悪いときに来合わせたかも，とドッキリしてしまい，何とあいさつしたものかと困りました．でもご本人は全く頓着する気配がないので，これまたびっくり！

この経験からは，欧米人は日本人よりもドライでオープンであるように見えます．でもこんな話もありました．

同じアメリカで，あるナースがクリニックの電話を前に思案していたそうです．担当の慢性病患者が来院しないので気になるのですが，自宅に電話をかけてみようか，いや自発的な受診を待つべきか，というのが彼女の悩みでした．

日本なら「お薬切れてますね，受診したらどうですか？」と専門職が電話をかければ，なんて親切な人だと言われるに違いありません．でも，自立の原則が何よりも尊重される社会では，担当ナースの一方的な親切は自立を侵すことになりかねません．

やはり外国人相手にはプライバシーってむずかしい！？

************** 応用フレーズ ***************

以前に手術をしたことがありますか	Have you ever had any operations?
手術をしたのは何歳の時ですか	How old were you when you had the operation?
以前になぜ入院されたのですか	Why were you hospitalized before?
最後にお風呂に入ったのはいつですか	When did you last take a bath?
どんな運動やスポーツをなさっていますか	What kinds of exercise or sports do you engage in?
宗教上受けられない治療はありますか	Is there any treatment you cannot undergo for a religious reason?

少し頭痛がします	I have a slight headache.
ひどい頭痛がします	I have a bad（terrible）headache.
偏頭痛がします	I have a migraine.
のぼせています	I fell the blood rushing to my head.

のどがヒリヒリします	My throat is burning.
のどが渇いた感じです	My throat feels dry.
のどがいがらっぽい感じです	My throat feels dry and raw and scratchy.
声が出なくなったことがあります	I've lost my voice.
口内炎ができています	I have sores in my mouth.
歯が痛いです	I have a toothache.

胃がもたれます	My stomach feels heavy.
胸が焼けます	I have heartburn.
吐きました	I vomited.　　　　（I threw up.）
鼻水が出ます	I have a runny nose.
鼻がつまっています	I have a stuffy nose.

記憶がなくなってしまいました	I suffer from memory loss.
気を失って倒れました	I fainted.
何がどうなっているかわかりません	I feel disoriented.
ひきつけがおきました	I went into convulsions.

おりものが出ます	I have a discharge.
血液のかたまりが出ました	I've passed clots.
生理中です	I'm having my period.
生理が不規則です	My period is irregular.
つわりがあります	I am suffering from morning sickness.
肌があれています	I have rough skin.
むくみがあります	I have edema.
蚊にさされました	I got mosquito bites.
蜂にさされました	I got a bee sting.
物がぼんやり見えます	Things look dim.
物が二重に見えます	I see things double.
物がゆがんで見えます	Things look distorted.

◪ **'I'd like to ask you 〜'**（〜をお聞きしたいのですが）◪

　入院患者さんの基本的な情報を得ておくことは，ケアに大変必要なことです．しかし，患者さんのプライバシーに関わることがあり，非常にデリケートです．次のようなていねいな表現を心がけましょう．

　'If you don't mind, would you tell me 〜'（おさしつかえなければ〜を教えてください）
　'I'd like to ask you 〜'（〜をお聞きしたいのですが）

Unit 3　What is worrying you the most?
あなたの気がかりは何でしょうか

Talk 3

Ns : What seems to be the problem?
　　（なにか気になることがありますか）

Pt : My greatest concern is 'money.'
　　（一番気になるのはお金のことです）

Ns : Do you have health insurance?
　　（保険には入っていますか）

Pt : Yes, I have insurance in America.　I'm not sure if it covers overseas hospitalization.
　　（アメリカで1つ入りました．それが海外での入院にも使えるのか，覚えてないのです）

Ns : You should contact your agent as soon as possible.
　　（すぐ問い合わせた方がいいですね）

Pt : Yes, I will.
　　（私もそう思います）

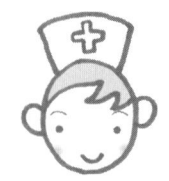

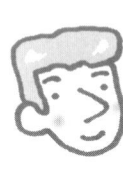

Lesson 3

Nurse

①何か困っていることがありますか	Are there any problems?
	Is anything wrong?
②何か問題はないですか	Is everything all right?
③どうかされました	Can I help you?
④大丈夫ですか．顔色が悪いですね	Are you all right? You look pale.
⑤前にもこういうことがありましたか	Have you had something like this before?
⑥よろしければ理由を教えていただけませんか	
	Will you tell me the reason, if you don't mind?
⑦相談にのってもらえるような親しい人がいますか	
	Do you have anyone close to you to consult?

Patient

⑧うちに帰りたい	I'd like to go home.
⑨ひとりぼっちだ	I'm lonely.
⑩退院はいつになるでしょうか	When will I be able to leave the hospital?
⑪治療費を見積もっていただけませんか	Could you calculate the fees?
⑫入院費が払えるかどうか心配です	I'm worrying about how to pay for the medical bills.
⑬家のことが気になって眠れません	
	I worry so much about my family that I can't sleep.
⑭傷跡は残りますか	Will there be a scar?
⑮友人に連絡が取れません	I can't contact my friend.
⑯英語がよくわかりません	I can't understand English well.
⑰通訳をたのめますか	Can I ask someone to interpret for me?
⑱何か大きな病気なのでしょうか	Am I seriously ill?
⑲長くかかるのでしょうか	Will it take a long time?
⑳いつ痛みがくるかと，不安です	I'm worried about getting the pain again.
㉑入院してから，便秘で困っています	
	I've had trouble with constipation since I entered the hospital.
㉒シャワーはいつでも使えますか	Can I use the shower any time?
㉓食事は毎食パンにすることができますか	Can I have bread at every meal?

Exercise 3

Listen to the CD and fill in the blanks.
（CDを聞いて，下線部分をうめなさい）

1. What is _____ you the most?
   （一番の気がかりは何ですか）
2. Please _____ _____ to ask me any questions.
   （どんなことでもきいて下さい）
3. Did you _____ the doctor's instructions?
   （先生の指示はわかりましたか）
4. I'm _____ I will get the severe pain again.
   （またひどく痛むのではないかと思います）
5. I'm very _____ .
   （非常に不安です）
6. I'm _____ _____ about my family.
   （一番の気がかりは家族のことです）
7. I'm so _____ .
   （たいへん孤独です）
8. After the divorce I sank into a deep _____ .
   （離婚後，ひどいうつ状態でした）
9. I sometimes feel like _____ _____ .
   （時々自殺したくなります）
10. I have no friend to _____ ____ .
    （相談できる友人がいません）

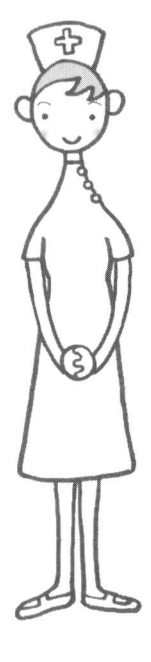

知っておきたい用語

1) 情緒不安定状態に関する用語

不安	anxíety	いらだち	irritátion
パニック	pánic	恐怖	fear
興奮	excítement	怒り	ánger
うつ状態	depréssion	躁状態	extréme enthúsiasm
対人恐怖	fear of other people	自意識	sélf-cónsciousness
自己尊重	sélf-estéem	自信喪失	sélf-distrúst
マタニティブルー	matérnity blues	更年期障害	menopáusal disórder
否認	deníal	絶望	despáir
疲労感	sense of fatígue	不眠（入眠困難）	insómnia
孤独	lóneliness	フラストレーション	frustrátion
無気力	léthargy	食欲不振	lack of áppetite
不信感	distrúst	過食	overéating
喪失	loss	悲嘆	grief

2) 現代社会の心の闇に関する用語

心的外傷体験	psychic trauma [sáikik tráuma]	アルコール依存	álcohol depéndence
燃えつき状態	búrn-out	薬物依存	drug depéndence
ドメスティックバイオレンス	doméstic víolence		
社会的孤立	sócial isolátion	閉じこもり	seclúsion
退行	degradátion	自殺企図	súicide attémpt
被害妄想	delúsion of persecútion	希死念慮	súicide feeling
誇大妄想	expánsive delúsion	虐待	abúse

3) ライフイベントに関する用語

結婚	márriage	再婚	remárriage
離婚	divórce	家族の増加	íncrease of fámily members
妊娠	prégnancy	就職	becoming emplóyed
子どもの独立	indepéndence of chíldren	卒業	graduátion
入学	starting school	転校	changing schools
引越し	move	配偶者の死	death of spouse
別居	separátion	近親者の死	death of kin

4) 社会的・家庭的諸要因に関する用語

昇進	promótion	上司とのトラブル	trouble with supériors
事業の開始	start of énterprise	退職	retírement
リストラ	dischárge	失業	únemplóyment
借金	debt	家のローン	loan to buy a house
病気・怪我	diséase, ínjury	交通事故	tráffic áccident
家族の病気	íllness of fámily member	家族の介護	care of fámily

『健康保険を活用しましょう』

　健康保険には，外国籍の人でも加入することができます．また，加入していれば，負担額やさまざまな公的医療福祉サービスの利用も，日本人と同じ条件です．つまり，難病等の特定疾患患者を対象にした医療費助成や，高額療養費払い戻し制度なども，同じ条件で適用される権利があります．

　しかし，日本での生活が浅く，とくに日本語の十分でない外国人の場合には，こういった制度について聞いたことのないことが多いものです．これらのサービスは申請する必要があるものが多く，また，申請が遅れた場合，さかのぼっての医療費補助は原則的になされません．

　せっかく加入していてもいざという時に活用できなかったということになりかねないのです．保険料を支払っている人が不利益をこうむることのないように，制度の運用についてナースもよく知っておく必要があるでしょう．大きな病院なら医療ケースワーカーが詳しい知識を持っています．健康保険制度についての問い合わせは，各市町村・区役所の国民健康保険課が担当しています．

　なお，健康保険への加入は外国人登録を済ませていることが条件で，在留資格のないいわゆるオーバーステイの状態では，健康保険への加入および生活保護の認定は非常に困難になります．このほか，外国人の未払い医療費補填（ほてん）制度があり，これは都道府県の事業です．

************ 応用フレーズ *************

入院を1週間遅らせることができますか　　Can the admission be put off for a week?
手術前に，髪を刈ることになるのでしょうか
　　　　　　　　　　　　　　　　　Must I have my hair cut before the operation?
いよいよ手術で緊張気味です
　　　　　　　　　　　　　　　It's almost time for the operation so I'm a bit nervous.
自己血輸血をお願いしたいのです
　　　　　　　　　　　　　　　　I'd like to receive an autologous blood transfusion.
手術のあと，どのくらいで歩けるようになるのでしょうか
　　　　　　　　　　　　　　　How long will it take to walk again after the operation?
副作用があるのにする価値があるのでしょうか
　　　　　　　　　　　　　　I wonder if it is worth trying in spite of the side effects.

これ，本当に痛み止めですか．全然効きません
　　　　　　　　　　　　　　　　Is this really a painkiller? It doesn't work at all.
眠いのは薬のせいでしょうか　　　Will this medicine make me sleepy?
吸入のあと，ずいぶん痰が出ます　I cough up a lot mucus after inhalation.
以前のように，食べたいという気持ちがわいてきません
　　　　　　　　　　　　　　　　　I don't have the appetite I used to have.
吐き気が続いて疲れています　　　I'm always feeling nauseated and exhausted.

院内に家族の泊まれるところはありますか
　　　　　　　　　　　　　　　　　Can my family stay overnight in the hospital?
院内からE-メールを送ることができますか
　　　　　　　　　　　　　　　　　Can I send my E-mail from this hospital?
心配なのは，妻の介護疲れです　　I'm afraid my wife will be exhausted.
フランス語で話せる人はいませんか　Is there anyone who can speak French?
アメリカに帰れば，もっといろいろな選択肢があると思うのです
　　　　　　　　　　　　　　　　I think I have more choices if I go back to America.

Unit 4

Let me show you around the ward.
病棟をご案内します

Talk 4

Ns : This sign shows the emergency escape route.
　　（この表示は避難経路を示しています）

Pt : You have many earthquakes here in Japan.
　　（日本は地震の多い国でしたね）

Ns : If a disaster should occur, a siren will sound.　There will also be announcements.
　　（災害発生時はサイレンが鳴ります．その旨アナウンスがあります）

Pt : Will the announcements be only in Japanese?
　　（アナウンスは日本語だけですか）

Ns : I'm sorry to say that the announcements will only be in Japanese.
　　（残念ながらそのとおりです）

Pt : That's too bad.
　　（それは困りますよ）

Ns : I'll discuss this with the head nurse.
　　（師長と相談しておきます）

◆　～をご案内します　◆

「病棟をご案内します」は 'I'll show you around the floor.' 'Let me show you around the floor.' どちらも使えますが，'Let me～' の方が「私にさせてください」のニュアンスがあります．

「病棟」にあたる英語は 'ward' です．でも多くの病院では階全体が一つの病棟になっている場合があります．例えば5階が全て小児病棟になっているような場合です．そのような場合は「病棟をご案内しましょう」と言うとき 'I'll show you around the floor.' というように 'floor'（階）を使ってもかまいません．しかし，一つの階に複数の病棟がある場合，'I'll show you around the floor.' と言うと他の病棟まで案内する事になってしまいますので，注意してください．

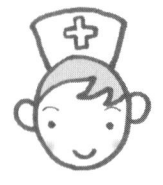

Lesson 4

①病室内をご説明しましょう	I'll show you your room.
②ロッカーはあそこです	The closet is over there.
③病棟をご案内しましょう	I'll show you around the ward.
	Let me show you around the ward.
④この手すりを使ってください	Hold onto the handrail.
⑤ナースステーションはこの先です	The nurse station is over there.
⑥ここのトイレは男性用です	This is the men's toilet.
⑦電気はここでつけます	The light switch is here.
⑧洗面所とトイレは分かれています	The washroom is separated from the lavatory.
⑨ここがお風呂です	This is the bath.
⑩この部屋へは入らないでください	This room is off limits.
⑪こちらのエレベーターをお使いください	Please use this elevator.
⑫売店は地下1階です．日用品を売っています	There is a store that sells sundries on the first basement floor.
⑬喫茶室は5階です	The coffee shop is on the fifth floor.
⑭喫煙コーナーは1階にあります	The smoking area is on the first floor.

『無意識下の差別はない？』

　ある中国籍の男性がケースワーカーに相談を希望しました．仕事中の事故で指を痛め，労災で入院していましたが，幸い障害も軽く退院もまぢかの人です．

　男性は中国籍でしたが，残留孤児の妻とともに日本滞在20年を超え，日本語には問題がありません．健康保険に加入しており，労災認定も受けていて，休業保険もおりていました．会社側の対応も手厚く，もし障害が残っても雇用は保証するといわれており，何も問題がないように見えました．

　男性が尋ねたのは，今回の様々なサービスに，「国籍による違いがあるか」ということでした．何か困ったので相談したというよりも，そのことを確認しておきたかったようです．担当したケースワーカーは，もちろん「何も違いはない」と請け合いました．医療費の計算式も示しました．それでも彼が納得して安心したかは結局わかりません．

　この男性がなぜあえて確認しておきたかったのか，どうしてなかなか安心できなかったのかには，複雑な背景があるに違いありません．公正な対応をしていると自信を持って説明できるか，ときどき改めて見直す必要もあるのでしょう．

Exercise 4

Listen to the CD and fill in the blanks.
（CDを聞いて，下線部分をうめなさい）

1. This is the _____ _____ .
   （こちらが洗濯室です）
2. This is the _____ _____ .
   （こちらがナースステーションです）
3. There are 20 _____ in this ward.
   （この病棟には病室が20室あります）
4. I'll show you the _____ _____ .
   （食堂をご案内しましょう）
5. You can meet your visitors in the _____ _____ .
   （談話室で面会に来られた方とお会いになって結構です）
6. You can go out from the _____ _____ .
   （この非常口から出てください）
7. Your child can play in the _____ _____ here.
   （お子さんはプレイルームで遊んでもらってください）
8. Here is the _____ _____ . You can push it any time.
   （こちらがナースコールです．いつでも押してください．）
9. Your visitors can smoke in the _____ _____ .
   （面会の方には喫煙所でたばこをすっていただいてください）
10. This is a _____ _____ . You can move here, if you pay an additional fee.
    （こちらが個室です．差額ベッド代をお支払いいただければ
    移っていただけます）

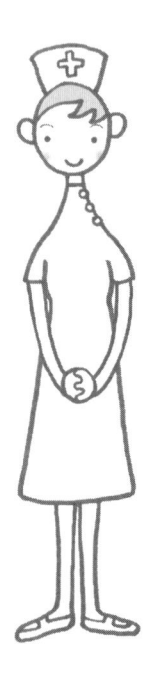

| 知っておきたい用語 |

1) 施設名
(病棟内)

病棟	ward	病室	hóspital room
個室	prívate room	食堂	díning room
洗面所	réstroom, báthroom	風呂場	báthroom
洗濯室	láundry room	コインランドリー	coin láundry
ナースステーション	núrse station	診察室	consultátion room
処置室	tréatment room	談話室	pátients' lounge
会議室	staff cónference room	喫煙所	smóking area
非常口	emérgency éxit	プレイルーム（小児科病棟内）	pláy room

(病棟外)（外来についての施設名については Unit 13 を見てください）

医局	dóctors' óffice	看護部	núrsing depártment
手術室	operátion room	回復室	recóvery room
集中治療室	inténsive care únit（ICU）		
冠状動脈疾患集中治療室	córonary care únit（CCU）		
周産期センター	perinátal cénter	新生児室	núrsery
分娩室	delívery room	伝染病棟	contágious diséase ward
救急病棟	emérgency ward		
図書室	líbrary		

2) 病院で働く人々　　　Hospital personnel

病院管理職　　administrator

| 院長 | hóspital diréctor | 副院長 | vice diréctor |
| 看護部長 | superinténdent of núrses | 事務長 | chief admínistrator |

医師　doctor

| 医師（スタッフ） | doctor, physícian | 研修医 | resident |

看護部　nursing depártment

看護部長	superinténdent of nurses
管理師長	súpervisor
病棟師長	head nurse（米）síster（英）
専門看護師	clínical nurse spécialist（CNS）

看護師	régistered nurse（R.N.）		
准看護師	lícensed práctical nurse（L.P.N.）		
看護助手	núrse's aide		
看護実習生	stúdent nurse		
薬剤師	phármacist	栄養士	dietítian, nutrítionist
理学療法士	phýsical thérapist	作業療法士	occupátional thérapist
言語療法士	speech thérapist	臨床心理士	clínical psychólogist
音楽療法士	músic thérapist	ソーシャルワーカー	médical sócial wórker
臨床検査技師	lab technícian	X線技師	X-ray technícian
視能訓練士	orthóptist		
歯科衛生士	déntal hýgienist	歯科技工士	déntal technícian
事務職員	clerk	会計係	cashíer
受付係	recéptionist	電話交換手	óperator
ボランティア	voluntéer		

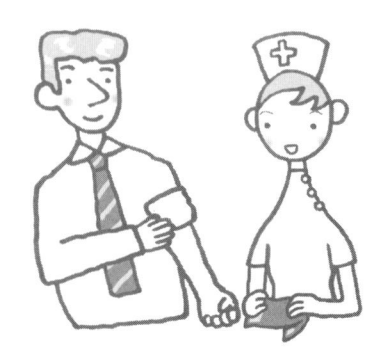

Floor Information

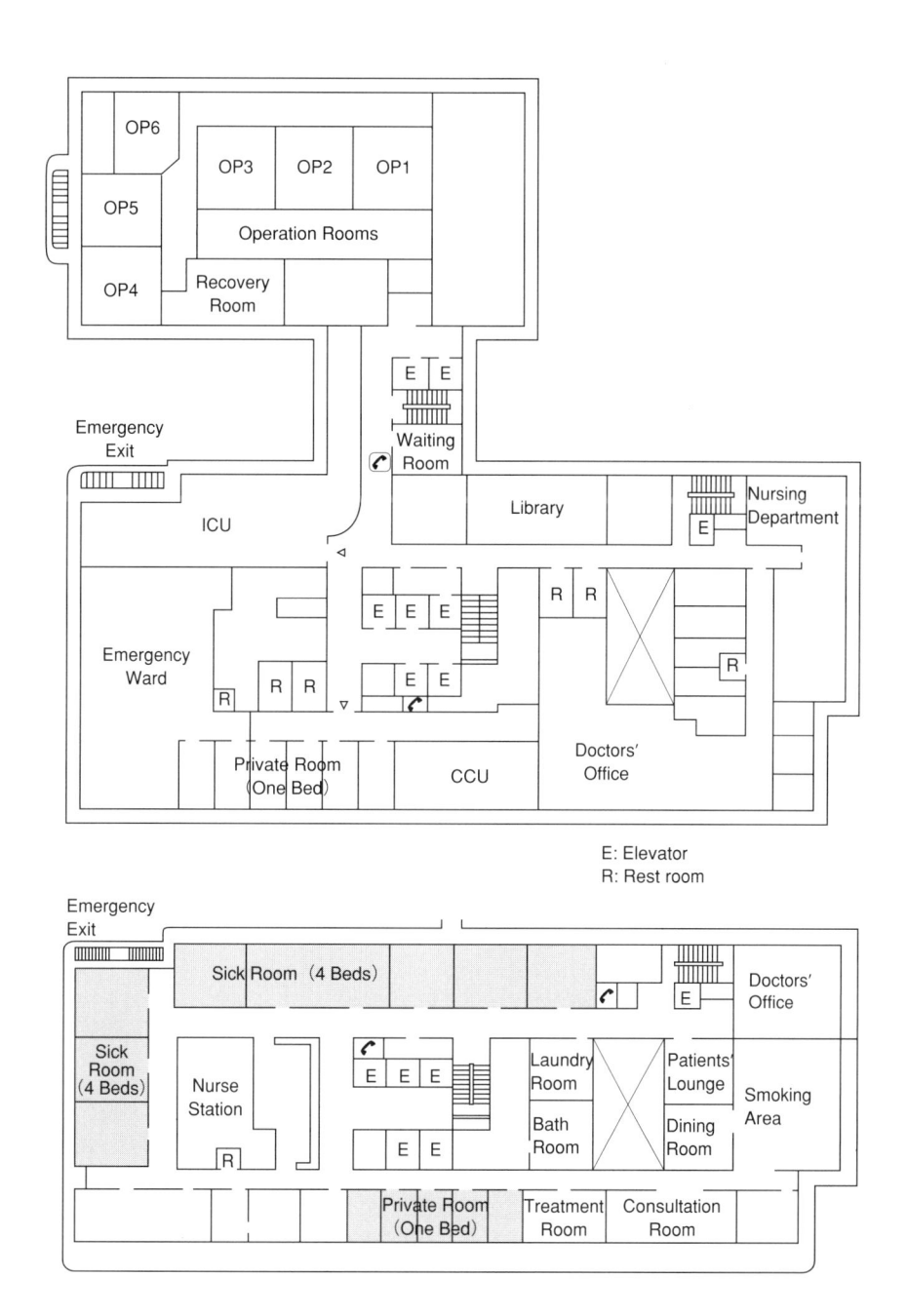

(Top floor plan)
- OP6, OP5, OP4, OP3, OP2, OP1 — Operation Rooms
- Recovery Room
- Emergency Exit
- Waiting Room
- ICU
- Library
- Nursing Department
- Emergency Ward
- Private Room (One Bed)
- CCU
- Doctors' Office

E: Elevator
R: Rest room

(Bottom floor plan)
- Emergency Exit
- Sick Room (4 Beds)
- Sick Room (4 Beds)
- Nurse Station
- Laundry Room
- Bath Room
- Patients' Lounge
- Dining Room
- Smoking Area
- Doctors' Office
- Private Room (One Bed)
- Treatment Room
- Consultation Room

（神戸市立西市民病院案内図をもとに作成）

Unit 5

Let's make a care plan.
ケアプランを立てましょう

Talk 5

Ns : I'm in charge of your care plan.
（私がケアプランを担当します）

Pt : What's a care plan?
（ケアプランとはどういうものですか）

Ns : It is to guide the nurses in taking care of the patient. Here is the care plan we have prepared for you.
（ナースが患者さんをお世話するためのプランです．こちらが入院中のケアプランです）

Pt : OK. Let me read it carefully before asking you questions about it.
（OK．質問する前によく読ませてください）

Ns : You will have several kinds of tests before the operation.
（手術前にいくつかの検査を受けてもらいます）

Pt : When will I be able to sit up after the operation?
（術後どのくらいで起き上がれるようになれますか）

Ns : In two or three days.
（2～3日です）

Pt : I see. Can I be back at work in two weeks?
（わかりました．2週間で職場復帰できますか）

Ns : That's up to you.
（あなた次第です）

◆ 'That's up to you.'（あなた次第です）◆

この表現は日本人には少し冷たく聞こえるかもしれませんが，英語圏の人は独立心が強く 'That's up to you.' と言われると発奮して治ろうとする気持ちが強くなる場合が多いです．この表現で患者さんを上手に励ますこともケアには必要でしょう．

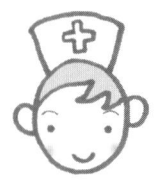

Lesson 5

Nurse

① 手術は今月の27日の予定です
　　You will have the operation on the 27th of this month.
② 毎朝8時に血圧を測ります　　We check blood pressure at 8 o'clock every morning.
③ 手術までに検査がいくつかあります
　　You have to go through several examinations before the operation.
④ 頭を少し剃らなければなりません　　We have to shave a portion of your head.
⑤ 腹式呼吸の練習をしましょう　　Let's practice abdominal breathing.

⑥ 手術の前日は絶食です　　You cannot eat on the day before the operation.
⑦ 手術の前日は流動食になります　　You will have a liquid diet on the day before surgery.
⑧ 明日から普通食になります　　You will have a regular diet from tomorrow on.
⑨ 毎日歩行訓練をすると早く治ります
　　You can get well sooner by practicing walking every day.
⑩ 手術翌日から歩いて構いません　　You can walk on the day after the operation.
⑪ 術後リハビリが必要です　　You will need rehabilitation after the operation.
⑫ 今から2週間で退院できます　　You can leave the hospital two weeks from now.

Patient

⑬ 手術日はいつですか　　When will I have the operation?
⑭ 毎日検査があるのですか　　Will I have the tests every day?
⑮ このケアプランのここはできそうもありません
　　I'm afraid I can't follow this care plan.
⑯ どうしてもタバコが吸いたいのですが　　I want to smoke very badly.
⑰ いつからタバコを吸ってかまいませんか　　When will I be able to start smoking?
⑱ 先生のご説明の際は家族の立会いも必要ですか
　　Does my family have to be present when the doctor gives the explanation?

Exercise 5

Listen to the CD and fill in the blanks.
（CDを聞いて，下線部分をうめなさい）

1. We will try _____.
   （放射線療法を使います）
2. You will have the _____ _____ every day during your hospitalization.
   （入院中，毎日糖尿病食です）
3. Please take a bath the day before the _____.
   （手術の前日にお風呂に入っていただきます）
4. We must _____ your chest to prepare you for the operation.
   （手術のために胸の毛を剃らなければなりません）
5. Will I receive _____ _____ after the operation?
   （手術のあと理学療法を受けることがあるのですか）
6. Who will make the _____ _____?
   （ケアプランは誰が立てるのですか）
7. Can I have a _____ _____?
   （普通食を食べられるのでしょうか）
8. Do I have to use the _____ after the operation?
   （術後はしびんを使わなければならないのでしょうか）
9. What is _____ _____?
   （腹式呼吸というのは何ですか）
10. How long will the _____ take?
    （リハビリが終わるまでにどのぐらいかかりますか）

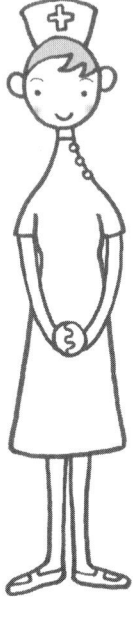

知っておきたい用語

1) 主な治療

外科的治療	súrgical thérapy	内科的治療	consérvative thérapy
食餌療法	aliméntothérapy	薬物治療	medícinal thérapy
化学療法	chémothérapy	放射線療法	rádiothérapy
臓器移植	órgan tránsplantátion	遺伝子治療	gene thérapy
理学療法	phýsical thérapy	作業療法	occupátional thérapy
言語療法	speech thérapy		

2) 食事用語

普通食	régular díet	減塩食	low salt díet
流動食	líquid díet	糖尿病食	diabétic díet
経管栄養	tube féeding	心臓病食	cárdiac díet
粥	(rice) grúel	離乳食	baby food
母乳	móther's milk, breast milk	母乳栄養	breast feeding
		人工栄養	artifícial feeding

3) 病室で使う器具・用具

電動ベッド	electromótive bed	オーバーベッドテーブル	over bed table
ナースコール	call button, call bell	洗面台	sink
酸素プラグ差込口	óxygen óutlet	冷蔵庫	refrígerator
ロッカー	clóset	ごみ箱	rúbbish can
床頭台	bédside table	懐中電灯	fláshlight
寝具一式	bédding	ゴム布	rubber sheet
マットレス	máttress	電気毛布	eláctric blánket
ふとん	quilt, cómforter		
洗面器	wash básin	病衣	hóspital gown
入れ歯	false teeth	下着	únderwear
衣類	clóthing	おむつ	díaper
パジャマ	pajámas	洗濯物	láundry

4) 看護用品

氷枕（ひょうちん）	ice píllow	しびん	úrinal
湯たんぽ	hot water bottle	便器	béd-pan
円座	rúbber air bag	眼帯	eye patch
点滴用ポール	intravénous injéction（IV）pole		
車いす	whéelchair	紙オムツ	paper díaper
松葉つえ	a pair of crútches		

「複雑な内容も分ければ簡単」

　ケアプランを立てることは，患者さんと一緒に，同じ目標に向かって努力する関係を作ることでもあります．現実的な見通しをもって，患者さんの状態に合った計画を立てるなかでは，こんな表現も必要になるでしょう．
　「明日の検査結果がよければ，お風呂に入りましょう」
　「1錠飲んで，まだ痛みが続くようなら，もう1錠飲みましょう」
　このような「もし〜なら…しましょう」といった条件を含む表現は，患者さん自身があらかじめ見通しをもったり，自分で様子を見ながら調整したりするときには欠くことができません．でもこれらの日本語をひとまとめに英語にしようとすると，構文が複雑になり，難しいですね．難しいと感じるとおっくうになるものです
　こういうときには内容のまとまりによって短く分けて表現してみましょう．

　Let's see the result of the test tomorrow. If they are OK, then you can take a bath.
　（明日の検査結果を見てみましょう．もしよければお風呂に入りましょう）
　Take one tablet. See if the pain stops. If the pain does not stop, then take one more tablet.
　（1錠飲みましょう．痛みが止まるか見てみましょう．もしとまらなければもう1錠飲みましょう）

　複雑な内容でも，このように短く区切ってみると，単純な文章の組み合わせで表現できる場合が多いものです．ふだんから意識してみませんか？

************** 応用フレーズ ***************

腹式呼吸は傷口への影響が少ない呼吸法です
　　　　　　　　　　　　　　　Abdominal breathing has a lesser effect on the wound.
カモードを使ってみませんか　　　How about using a commode chair?
カモードというのは洋式の室内用トイレです
　　　　　　　　　　　　　　　A commode chair is a kind of chair with a chamber-pot.
ガスが出るまでお水は飲めません　You can't drink water until you have passed gas.
熱がある時はお風呂に入れません　You can't take a bath when you have a fever.
血圧を下げるために塩分を控えた食事が必要です
　　　　　　　　　　　　　　　You need a low salt diet to reduce your blood pressure.
手術の前は，髪を切らなければなりません
　　　　　　　　　　　　　　　We have to cut your hair before the operation.

手術のためにしておかなければならないことがありますか
　　　　　　　　　　　　　　　Is there anything I have to do to prepare for the operation?
このケアプランは変えていただきたいです　I'd like to change the care plan.

◘ 'I hope〜'　（そうなるといいですね）◘

　'You will be able to walk in a month.' というような表現をした場合，実際そのことが実現できない場合もあり，そのときには患者さんをがっかりさせてしまいます．この場合 'I hope を前につけて 'I hope you will be able to walk in a month.'（1ヶ月で歩けるようになるといいですね）とすると，ナースと一緒に頑張りましょうという気持ちもこもるので，とても良い表現になります．

　一方，良くないことも伝えなければならない場合があります．'You will have some pain tomorrow.' というような表現をした場合，とても冷たく患者さんを傷つけてしまう場合もあります．この場合はI'm afraid を前につけて 'I'm afraid you will have some pain tomorrow.'（残念ながら明日も痛みがあると思います）というようにすると和らいだ表現になります．

　'I hope' 'I'm afraid' を知っていると，随分幅広いコミュニケーションが可能になります．上手に使ってみましょう．

Unit 6

What is 'informed consent'?
「インフォームドコンセント」って何ですか

Talk 6

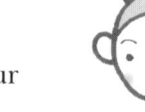

Ns : Has the doctor-in-charge informed you about your therapy?
（主治医から治療法についての説明は受けられましたか）

Pt : Yes.　There are several choices of therapy.
（はい，治療の選択肢はいくつかあるようです）

Ns : What kind of therapy have you decided on?
（どの治療法に決められたのですか）

Pt : I've decided to receive chemotherapy.
（化学療法を受けることにしました）

Ns : Were you satisfied with the explanation?
（よく納得されたのですね）

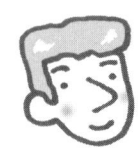

Pt : Yes. The doctor informed me about each possible treatment in detail.　I could understand the explanations very well.
（はい．先生はそれぞれの治療法について詳しく説明してくださいましたのでよく理解できました）

Lesson 6

Nurse

① 病状について医師から明日説明したいのですが
　　　　　　　　　　　　　　The doctor will talk to you about your illness tomorrow.
② 手術について先生から説明があります
　　　　　　　　　　　　　　The doctor is going to explain the operation to you.
③ 承諾書はよく読みましたか　　　Have you read the consent form carefully?
④ 先生が先ほど説明された承諾書です
　　　　　　　　　　　　　　This is the consent form the doctor told you about.
⑤ 主治医からの説明は理解できましたか
　　　　　　　　　　　　　　Could you understand what the physician-in-charge said?
⑥ 先生にお聞きになりたいことはありませんか
　　　　　　　　　　　　　　Is there anything you would like to ask the doctor?
⑦ 専門用語が難しくありませんか　Did you find the technical terms difficult?

Patient

⑧ 主治医の先生にお話したいことがあるのですが
　　　　　　　　　　　　　　I'd like to talk with my physician.
⑨ また先生にご相談したいことがでてきました
　　　　　　　　　　　　　　I'd like to consult the doctor about another problem.
⑩ 先生とアポイントメントをとりたいのですが
　　　　　　　　　　　　　　I'd like to make an appointment with the physician.
⑪ 考える時間を少しください　　　I'd like to have some time to think about it.
⑫ 先生の言われたことに同意できません　I can't consent to the doctor's suggestion.
⑬ 放射線療法を受けることにしました　I've decided to receive radiotherapy.

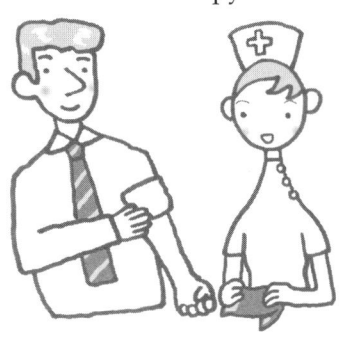

Exercise 6

Listen to the CD and fill in the blanks.
(CDを聞いて，下線部分をうめなさい)

1. Did you understand the doctor's explanation of the _____ _____?
   (先生の副作用の説明はおわかりになりましたか)
2. Have you signed the _____ _____?
   (承諾書のサインされましたか)
3. Did you understand the explanation about the condition of your _____?
   (糖尿病の状態についての説明はおわかりになりましたか)
4. Are you planning to go back to the United States for your _____?
   (アメリカに帰られて治療することを考えておられるのですか)
5. Could you understand the _____ _____?
   (専門用語はおわかりになりましたか)
6. I haven't decided on the _____ yet.
   (まだ治療について決めていません)
7. The doctor explained to me about the condition of my _____.
   (先生が肺炎について説明してくださいました)
8. I _____ _____ the operation.
   (手術に同意します)
9. I have more _____ for the doctor.
   (さらに先生にお聞きしたい事があります)
10. I cannot decide on whether to consent to the _____.
    (手術の決心がつきません)

知っておきたい用語

1) 消化器系疾患

胃炎	gastrítis	胃潰瘍	gástric úlcer
胃がん	stómach cáncer		stómach úlcer
肝炎	hepatítis	肝硬変	líver cirrhósis
肝臓がん	líver cáncer	大腸がん	cólon cáncer
直腸がん	réctal cáncer	虫垂炎（盲腸炎）	appendicítis
食中毒	food póisoning		

2) 循環器系疾患

心臓病	heart diséase	心臓発作	heart attáck
心不全	heart fáilure	心筋梗塞	myocárdial infárction
高血圧症	hyperténsion	狭心症	angína

3) 呼吸器系疾患

肺炎	pneumónia	肺がん	lung cáncer
結核	tuberculósis（TB）	気管支炎	bronchítis
喘息	ásthma		

4) 腎・尿路疾患

膀胱炎	cystítis	腎炎	nephrítis
ネフローゼ	nephrósis	前立腺癌	próstate cáncer

5) 代謝疾患

糖尿病	diabétes	痛風	gout
バセドー氏病	Básedow's diséase		

6) 血液疾患

貧血	anémia	白血病	leukémia
血友病	hemophília		

7) 骨・関節疾患

骨折	frácture	脱臼	dislocátion
ねんざ	sprain	関節炎	arthrítis
骨粗鬆症	osteoporósis	リューマチ	rhéumatism

8) 感染症

はしか	méasles	風疹	rubélla
おたふく風邪	mumps	インフルエンザ	flu（inflúenza）
マラリア	malária	コレラ	chólera

エイズ（後天性免疫不全症候群）		AIDS (Acquired Immunodeficiency Sýndrome)	

9) 脳・神経疾患

脳卒中	stroke	脳腫瘍	brain túmor
パーキンソン病	Párkinson's diséase	痴呆	deméntia
老人性痴呆	sénile deméntia	アルツハイマー病	Álzheimer's diséase
脳動脈瘤	áneurysm		

10) 精神疾患

精神分裂病	schizophrénia	心身症	psychosomátic disórder
躁病	mánia	うつ病	depréssion
不眠症	insómnia	ヒステリー症	hystéria
ノイローゼ	neurósis	不安神経症	anxíety neurósis
神経性食欲不振症	anoréxia nervósa		

11) その他

乳がん	breast cáncer	子宮筋腫	úterine myóma
子宮癌	úterine cáncer		
花粉症	hay féver	扁桃炎	tonsillítis
白内障	cátaract	緑内障	glaucóma
トラホーム	trachóma	結膜炎	conjunctivítis
皮膚がん	skin cáncer	やけど	burn
じんましん	hives	にきび	ácne
水虫	áthlete's foot	わきが	body ódor
あせも	heat rash	いぼ	wart

************** 応用フレーズ **************

手術が延期できるか，先生に相談してみますか
　　　　　　　　　Will you ask the doctor if we can put off the operation?
外来が済んだ後に，来てもらえるように医師に話しておきます
　　　　　　　　　I'll ask the doctor to come after consultation hours.
どこで治療されるかは，あなたが決められたらいいことです
　　　　　　　　　You can decide yourself where you'll receive the treatment.
承諾書にサインしてください．先生にお渡ししておきます
　　　　　　　　　Please sign the consent form.　I'll give it to the doctor.

説明されたことが理解できませんでしたが，先生には言いませんでした．
     I could not understand what the doctor was saying but I didn't say so.
アメリカでは，もっといろいろな選択肢があることを先生に教えていただきました．
     The doctor told me I would have more choices in the United States.

『インフォームドコンセント』

 Informed consentは日本語でもインフォームドコンセントという言葉が使われるようになっていますが，「説明と同意」と訳されることもあります．この英語はinformed（知らされた）consent（同意），すなわち，「病状について充分説明をうけ，その上で治療方法等について同意すること」です．

 カルテ開示などが当然になっているアメリカでは，患者さんによく納得のいく説明をした上で，治療方針の同意を得ることが必要です．

 日本では，「医師にお任せする」というような表現があるように，医師に説明を求めず，全てを任せるという風土がありました．家父長制度が長く続いた日本では，父親が家族全体を支配していましたが，そのかわり，家族全体を守るという責任も持っておりました．これと同様，医師も患者さんにあまり説明はせず，自分の責任において治療をしていました．このような父親や医師に見られる姿勢を'paternalistic attitude'（家父長のような姿勢）と呼んでいます．また医療での慣習を'medical paternalism'と呼んでいます．

 Informed consentとは本来 informed choice でなければなりません．すなわち複数の治療法から患者さん自身が選択できなくてはならないのです．アメリカでは，子供のころから，様々なことを自分が「選択する」という教育，トレーニングを受けていますので，治療を受ける場合も「選択」できなければ，フラストレーションを起こしてしまいます．アメリカではinformed choiceは当然なのです．医事訴訟の多いアメリカ社会では，ドクターにとっても患者さんがinformed choiceができる状況を作っておくことは大切なことです．だからナースも説明責任があるし，いろいろ聞かれることを覚悟しておかなくてはなりません．

 日本では，アメリカのように自分で「選択する」習慣がありません．病気のときにいきなり「選択してください」と言われても困ってしまいます．日本人には「説明と同意」―「一応説明してもらって，（自分で選択せずに）同意する」ことの方が合っているようです．

 このように文化が違うと，随分状況が違ってきます．ナースもケアをきちんと説明して，同意を得てから行うのは同じですよ．

Unit 7

What kind of pain is it?
どのように痛みますか

Talk 7

Ns : I hear you have a headache.　When did it start?
　　（頭が痛いそうですね．いつからですか）

Pt : It started about 30 minutes ago.
　　（30分くらい前からです）

Ns : Does your whole head ache or a part of it?
　　（痛いのは頭全体ですか　それとも部分的ですか）

Pt : My whole head.
　　（頭全体です）

Ns : What kind of pain is it?　Is it a griping pain?
　　（どのように痛みますか　きりきりとした鋭い痛みですか）

Pt : No. It's a dull pain as if I got hit on the head.
　　（違います．殴られた後のような鈍い痛みです）

Ns : It may be a side effect of your medicine.　I'll call the doctor.
　　（薬の副作用かもしれませんね．ドクターを呼んできます）

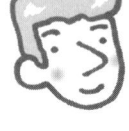

◆　「痛いよ！」　◆

「痛いっ！」という叫び声には 'Ouch' 'Ow' 'Ahh' 'Ooooo' などがあります．'Ouch' 'Ow' は一瞬痛いとき，'Ahh' 'Ooooo' はずーっと痛いときに使います．

「〜が痛い」という場合，前置詞 'in' を使って次のように言います．覚えておくと便利です．

I have a pain in the chest.
I have a throbbing pain in my arm.
I'm suffering from a pain in the chest.

Lesson 7

Nurse

① 痛みますか 　　　　　　　　　Do you have a pain?
　　　　　　　　　　　　　　　　Are you in pain?

② どのような痛みですか 　　　　What kind of pain do you have?
　　　　　　　　　　　　　　　　What kind of pain is it?
　　　　　　　　　　　　　　　　Could you describe the pain?

③ どこが痛みますか 　　　　　　Where does it hurt?
④ いつから痛みましたか 　　　　When did the pain start?
⑤ どのくらいの時間痛んでいますか　How long have you had the pain?
⑥ どういう時に痛みますか 　　　When do you feel the pain?
⑦ 痛そうですね 　　　　　　　　You seem to be in pain.
⑧ 大丈夫ですか 　　　　　　　　Are you all right?

Patient

⑨ ちくちくする痛みがあります 　I have a prickling pain.
⑩ 頭がずきずきします 　　　　　I have a throbbing headache.
⑪ 少し痛みます 　　　　　　　　It hurts a little.
⑫ ここがずきずきします 　　　　I have a throbbing pain here.
⑬ 間をおいて痛みがあります 　　It hurts on and off.
⑭ さわると痛みます 　　　　　　It hurts when I touch it.
⑮ 座っていられません 　　　　　I can't sit still.
⑯ 痛みがひどくて眠れません 　　It hurts so much that I can't sleep.
⑰ 息が止まりそうになります 　　I almost have to stop breathing.
⑱ この痛みを止めてください 　　Please stop this pain.
⑲ 今は治っています 　　　　　　I'm OK now.

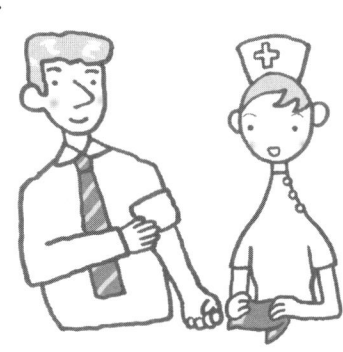

Exercise 7

Listen to the CD and fill in the blanks.
（CDを聞いて，下線部分をうめなさい）

1. Do you _____ _____ _____ when you walk?
   （歩くと痛いですか）
2. When do you have a _____ _____?
   （どんな時に軽い痛みがありますか）
3. Could you describe your _____?
   （どのように胃が痛いですか）
4. How long will it take for the _____ to _____?
   （痛みが治まるまでにどのぐらいの時間がかかります）
5. How _____ is the joint _____?
   （関節痛の痛みの強さはどのくらいですか）
6. I have a _____ _____ here.
   （ここがきりきりします）
7. The pain stops soon after I take a _____.
   （痛み止めを飲むとすぐに痛みは止まります）
8. It _____ when I press it.
   （押すと痛みます）
9. What should I do to _____ the pain?
   （痛みを和らげるのにはどうすればいいのですか）
10. I wake up because of the _____ pain.
    （うずくような痛みで何度も目がさめます）

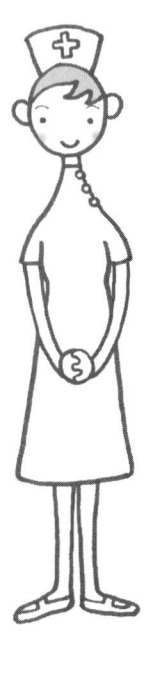

知っておきたい表現

1) 痛みのいろいろな表現

ちくちくする痛み	príckling pain（stábbing pain）
ずきずきする痛み	thróbbing pain
きりきり（しくしく）する痛み	gríping pain
ぎゅっとくる痛み	squéezing pain
刺すような痛み	stínging pain
焼けるような（ひりひりする）痛み	búrning pain
差し込むような痛み	cútting pain
激しい痛み	sharp pain
ひどい痛み	sevére pain
うずくような痛み	shóoting pain
耐えられない痛み	intráctable pain
ちょっとした痛み	slight（mild）pain
鈍痛	dull pain, áche
急性の痛み	acúte pain
慢性の痛み	chrónic pain
断続的な痛み	intermíttent pain
絶え間ない痛み	contínuous pain
しつこい痛み	persístent pain
局部的な痛み	lócalized pain
広範囲にわたる痛み	géneralized pain
しびれるような痛み	númbness

2) ～痛 があります（します）　　I have a ＿＿＿.

頭痛がします	I have a héadache.
胃痛がします	I have a stómachache.
腰痛があります	I have a lumbago.
関節が痛みます	I have a joint pain.

◆　身体の各部の痛み　◆

身体各部の痛みを表す語には次の3つのパターンがあります．

〜acheは慢性的な痛みの意味あいがあります．

〜painは一般的なすべての痛みに使われます．

1)「体の部位」＋ache

頭痛	headache	耳痛	earache
歯痛	toothache	胃痛	stomachache

2)「体の部位」＋pain　（学術用語では　+algia　または　+odynia）

頸部痛	neck pain	trachelodynia
筋肉痛	muscle pain	myalgia
腹痛	abdominal pain	celialgia
胸部痛（総称名）	chest pain	

3) それ以外

腰痛	lumbago	けいれん痛	cramp
圧迫痛	pressure	偏頭痛	migraine
のど（咽頭）痛	sore throat		

『Painがないだけでなく』

痛みへの対処は，ナースにとってもっとも力を注ぐところのひとつでしょう．ところで，痛みといえばpainが真っ先に頭に浮かびますが，英語でpainという言葉が使われるのは，かなり輪郭のはっきりした限局的な強い痛みが多いようです．

訴えをよく聞いていると，「なにか変だ」「ちょっと辛い」といったとき，患者さんはpainよりもsoreをしきりに使う，とあるナースが教えてくれました．患者さん自身がこれは痛みだとはっきりとらえている 'I have a pain' にくらべて，soreはそこが気になってどうにも落ち着かない，ひりひりして思わず手をそえたくなるような，より肌感覚に近い言葉のようです．'Sore foot' 'Sore head' 'Sore throat' といった身体のことにも，'She is sorely missing him.' のような心のことにも使われます．

ナースは，患者さんが「painがあるから薬をください」と言うかなり前に，患者さんのようすから（痛いのかな？）と気がつく場合が多いでしょう．そういうときには 'Is it sore?' または 'Does it hurt?' と声をかけてみます．なんとかしてくれと訴えるほどではなくとも，ナースが関心を向けることで患者さんも話しやすくなります．

また，尋ねてみたことで，痛みの原因になっている異変が早い時期に特定され，事態が悪化する前に対処できるかもしれません．

こうしてみると，ナースは単にpainがあるかないかに目を向けているだけでなく，それ以前の不快や居心地の悪さ，辛さへも敏感に気づいていこうと努力していることにあらためて気がつきますね．

************ 応用フレーズ **************

夜も痛みで目がさめますか	Do you wake up at night because of the pain?
だんだんひどくなっていますか．軽くなっていますか	Has the pain got severer or milder?
痛みのない状態を0，一番強い痛みを10とすると，今の痛みはいくつでしょうか	The painless condition is 0, the severest one is 10. How much is the pain you have now?
痛みの様子をこの表に記録してください	Please record your pain here on this chart.
いつも痛いというわけではないのですね	You don't always have a pain?
痛みがとれれば，もっとやる気になれますよ	When the pain has gone, you can be more active.
いつも深夜に痛くなるようですね	You always have a pain in the middle of the night. Is that right?
痛くなったら飲むように言われている薬があります	I have the medicine to take in case of pain.
痛み止めを飲んだことを記録してください	Please keep a record of when you take a painkiller.
痛み止めの量と時間を検討してみましょう	We'll review the dosage and time to take the painkiller.
気の休まるときがないのですね	You always feel anxious.
効き目の速い痛み止めを使うことができます	You can take a painkiller which will have an immediate effect.
痛みがひどくなる前に飲むとこの薬はよく効きます	The medicine works well before the pain gets severe.
痛みはひどくなったり，軽くなったりします	The pain becomes stronger and weaker.
痛みは徐々にきました	The pain came on slowly.
痛みは突然やってきました	The pain came on suddenly.
痛みの強い時間が長くなってきています	The length of time I am in severe pain has become longer.
いつ痛みがくるかと，不安です	I am worried that I'll be in pain again.
何かをしていると痛みを忘れます	I can forget about the pain when I'm doing something.
温めると痛みがおさまります	The pain stops when I am warm.

★☆★☆★☆★☆★☆★☆　人体各部の名称（1）　★☆★☆★☆★☆★☆★☆★

胃痛 stomachache，関節痛 joint pain は，体の部位を表す語に痛みを表す語が結びついて症状を表す言葉になります．このようなケースは医学用語にはたくさんあります．例えば，炎症を表す語（ear infection）や癌を表す語（lung cancer）などが結びついた病名にはよくお目にかかりますね．体の内部の主な用語を覚えておきましょう．体の外部の用語については Unit 9 を見てください．

1）骨格系

骨	bone		
頭蓋	skull	脊椎，背骨	spine
鎖骨	cóllarbone	胸骨	bréastbone
肋骨	rib	肩甲骨	shóulder blade
骨盤	pélvis		
大たい骨	fémur（pl. femora）	膝蓋骨，ひざ皿	knee cap
脊髄	spínal cord	骨髄	bone márrow

2）脳・神経系

脳	brain		
大脳	cerébrum	小脳	cerebéllum
神経	nerve		

3）筋・関節系

筋肉	múscle	腱	téndon
靭帯	lígament	関節	joint

4）呼吸器系

気管	tráchea	気管支	brónchi
肺	lung	胸郭	thórax
横隔膜	díaphragm		

5）循環器系

心臓	heart	血管	blood véssel
動脈	ártery	静脈	vein

血液	blood		
白血球	white blood cell, léukocyte		
赤血球	red blood cell, erýthrocyte		
リンパ	lymph	血清	sérum
リンパ球	lýmphocyte	リンパ腺	lymph gland

6) 口腔・消化器系

口腔	óral cávity	舌	tóngue
咽頭	phárynx	喉頭	lárynx
食道	esóphagus, gúllet	咽喉	throat
胃	stómach	十二指腸	duodénum
胆嚢	gall bládder	脾臓	spléen
膵臓	páncreas	肝臓	líver
小腸	small intéstine	空腸	jejúnum
回腸	íleum	大腸	cólon, large intéstine
上行結腸	ascénding cólon	横行結腸	transvérse cólon
下行結腸	descénding cólon	S状結腸	sígmoid cólon
盲腸	cécum	虫垂	appéndix
直腸	réctum	肛門	ánus

7) 泌尿器・生殖器系

腎臓	kídney	膀胱	bládder
尿道	uréthra		
生殖器	génitals	子宮	womb, úterus
膣	vagína	卵巣	óvary
睾丸	tésticle	陰茎	pénis
前立腺	próstate		

8) その他

瞳	púpil
涙腺	lácrimal gland
網膜	rétina
皮膚	skin
毛穴	póre

Unit 8

We'll do some tests.
検査をしましょう

Talk 8

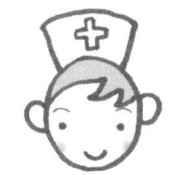

Ns : Let me take your blood pressure.　Please hold out your right arm.
　　（血圧を測りましょう．右腕を出していただけますか）

Pt : Like this?
　　（これでいいですか）

Ns : OK.　Please relax and take a deep breath.　Your arm feels tense.
　　（いいですよ．力を抜いて，深呼吸してください．腕が締まる感じがしますよ）

Pt : Is it high?
　　（高いですか）

Ns : It's 154 over 76.　It's a little bit lower than yesterday.
　　（154の76でした．昨日より少し低いですね）

Ns : Now let me take your temperature.　Please put the thermometer under your arm.
　　（次に体温を測りましょう．体温計を脇の下に挟んでください）

Pt : OK.
　　（はい）

Ns : Take out the thermometer when you hear the beeping sound.
　　（音が鳴ったら，体温計を出してくださいね）

Pt : I hear the beeping sound now.
　　（今鳴りましたよ）

Ns : It's 37.8 degrees Celsius.　You seem to have a slight fever.　It's higher than this morning.
　　（37度8分でした．少し熱がありますね．今朝より高いですね）

Lesson 8

〈尿検査　　urine test〉

Nurse

①尿検査をさせてください　　　　　Let me do a urine test.

②カップの1/3ぐらいまで尿を入れてください
　　　　　　　　　　　　　　　Please fill about one-third of the cup with urine.

③このコップに明日朝一番の尿を採ってください．
　　　　　　　　　　Please fill the cup when you first urinate tomorrow morning.

④最初の尿は捨てて，途中からのを採ってください
　　　　　　　　Please throw away the first portion of the urine, and take a sample
　　　　　　　　of the urine midway during urination.

⑤尿を入れたカップはトイレの棚においてください
　　　　　　　　　Leave the cup of urine on the designated shelf in the toilet.

⑥採尿ができたら教えてください　　Please let us know when you take your urine sample.

Patient

⑦尿はどのくらい採ればよいのでしょうか　　How much urine should I collect?

⑧尿が少ししか出ませんが　　　　I can pass only a little urine.

〈検便　　stool test〉

Nurse

⑨検便をさせてください　　　　　Let me do a stool test.

⑩便をこの容器に入れて持ってきてください
　　　　　　　　　　　　　　　Please bring a stool specimen in this container.

⑪このガラス棒を肛門に挿入し，取り出してください
　　　　　　　　　　　　Insert this glass stick into your rectum, and then take it out.

Patient

⑫便はどのくらい採ればよいでしょうか　　How much stool should I collect?

〈採血　　taking blood sample〉

Nurse

⑬血液検査をさせてください　　　Let me do a blood test.

⑭5 cc採血します　　　　　　　　I'm going to collect 5 cc.

⑮右手を出してください　　　　　　Please hold out your right arm.
⑯握りこぶしを作ってください　　　Please make a fist.
⑰チクとしますよ　　　　　　　　　This may hurt a little.
⑱力を抜いて楽にしてください　　　Please relax.
⑲3分間しっかりおさえていてください　Please press firmly for 3 minutes.
⑳気分が悪くなったら言ってください　Please let us know if you feel sick.
　　　　　　　　　　　　　　　　　（～ if you don't feel well.）

Patient
㉑何を調べるのですか　　　　　　　What are you going to test for?
㉒どのくらい血液を採るのですか　　How much blood are you going to collect?

〈血圧，脈，体温〉

Nurse
㉓血圧を計ります　　　　　　　　　Let me take your blood pressure.
　（脈，体温）　　　　　　　　　　（pulse, temperature）
㉔袖をまくってください　　　　　　Roll up your sleeve, please.
㉕ゆっくり息を吸って吐いてください　Please breathe in and out slowly.
㉖腋の下に汗をかいていますか　　　Are you sweating in your armpit?
㉗タオルで汗をふいてください　　　Please wipe away the sweat with the towel.

Patient
㉘何度でしたか　　　　　　　　　　What's my temperature?

　　　◆　摂氏と華氏　◆

　体温（温度）の単位には2種類あります．日本ではCentigrade（Celsius）（C）（摂氏）が使われていますが，アメリカ，イギリスでは主にFahrenheit（F）（華氏）が使われています．自分の平熱は96.8度（華氏）だと思っている患者さんが，突然「体温は36.0度です」（華氏96.8度＝摂氏36.0度）と言われたら驚いてしまいます．注意してください．

　摂氏と華氏の換算方法は次のようになります．
　　　華氏への換算　　$F = C \times \frac{9}{5} + 32$
　　　摂氏への換算　　$C = F - 32 \times \frac{5}{9}$

　なお摂氏36.0度は 'thirty-six degrees Celsius'，華氏96.8度は 'ninety-six point eight degrees Fahrenheit' と読みます．

Exercise 8

Listen to the CD and fill in the blanks.
（CDを聞いて，下線部分をうめなさい）

1. Pass a small amount of _____ into the toilet.
   （少しトイレに排尿してください）
2. I'm sorry but this is going to _____ a bit.
   （痛くしてごめんなさい）
3. Make a _____ like this.
   （このように握りこぶしを作ってください）
4. I'd like to check your condition. Let me take your blood pressure, _____ and _____ first.
   （あなたの状態を知りたいので先ず血圧，脈，体温を測らせてください）
5. Do you know what your _____ _____ is?
   （血圧はどのくらいかご存知ですか）
6. Your blood pressure is _____ _____ _____. It's normal.
   （血圧は　　で，正常です）
7. The _____ must stay under your arm for 3 minutes.
   （体温計は3分間腋の下にはさんでおかなければなりません）．
8. My temperature was _____ Celsius when I took it at home.
   （家で測った時は　　℃でした）
9. We would like to take _____ _____ to check your lungs.
   （肺を調べるために胸部写真を撮りましょう）
10. Have you had an _____ taken at another hospital?
    （他の病院でMRIを撮ったことがありますか）

知っておきたい用語

1) 検査に関する用語

呼吸器の検査

肺機能検査	púlmonary fúnction test（PFT）
肺活量検査	spirómeter test
喀痰検査	spútum examinátion
呼吸数	respirátion rate

循環器の検査

心電図	electrocárdiogram（ECG, EKG）
心臓カテーテル検査	cárdiac catheterizátion
造影剤	dye
バイタルサイン	vítal signs
不整脈	irrégular pulse

消化器の検査

胃カメラ検査	gastróscopy
大腸鏡検査	cólonoscopy
直腸バリウム検査	bárium énema examinátion
内視鏡検査	endóscopy

その他の検査用語

X線撮影	X́-ray
CTスキャン	compúter tomógraphy scan（CT）
磁気共鳴画像法	magnétic résonance ímaging（MRI）
ポジトロンCT, 陽電子放出断層撮影	pósitron emíssion tomógraphy（PET）
X線体軸断層撮影法	compúterized áxial tomógraphy（CAT）
超音波検査法	ultrasonógraphy（USG）

◧ **'Vital signs'**（バイタルサイン）◨

バイタルサインとは，生命徴候（脈拍・呼吸・体温など）のことで，これらを測ることは医療の基本です．現場では日本語でも「バイタルサイン」ということばを使っています．

日本語では，それぞれ「脈拍（呼吸・体温）を測らせてください」と言いますが，英語ではこれらをまとめて 'I'd like to take your vital signs.' といいます．

筋電図	electromýogram（EMG）
脳波	electroencéphalogram（EEG）
生検	bíopsy
細胞検査	cell análysis, tíssue cell análysis
肝機能検査	liver fúnction test

計測器具

体温計	thermómeter
血圧計	manómeter
駆血帯	tóurniquet
聴診器	stéthoscope
体重計	scale

医療検査機器

肺活量計	spirómeter
胃カメラ	gastrocámera
胃ファイバースコープ	fíberscope
内視鏡	éndoscope
気管支鏡	brónchoscope
腹腔鏡	láparoscope
24時間心電図モニター	24-hour Holter mónitor

◘　略号の読み方　◘

医療現場ではCT，MRI，ECG，EMG，EEG，USGのような頭文字をつないだ略号がたくさん出てきます．その呼称は，普通そのままアルファベット読みします．なお，母音が適宜入って1つの英単語のようになる場合，例えばPET，CATは［pet］［kæt］と読みます．

医療現場では速やかに対処しなければならないので，このように頭文字を使うことが非常に多いので覚えておきましょう．

このような頭字語のことを 'acronym' といいます．

*************** 応用フレーズ ***************

結果はいつわかりますか	When will I get the results?
結果は今日の午後わかります	You will have the results this afternoon.
尿が出ないときはお水を飲んで30分後にもう一度トライしてください	If you cannot urinate, drink water and try again after 30 minutes.
導尿をしましょう	Let's do the urethral catheterization.
トイレはどこですか	Where is the toilet?
あちらのトイレをお使いください	Use the toilet over there.
尿のカップをどこにおけばよいのでしょうか	Where should I leave the cup of urine?
親指をなかにして握ってください	Make a fist, with your thumb inside. Squeeze firmly, please.
痛いですか	Is it going to hurt?
痛いよ	You're hurting me. / That hurts!
脈が弱いみたいで心配です	I'm worried because my pulse is weak.
血圧は正常です	Your blood pressure is normal.

◆　便利な 'take' と 'do'　◆

血圧（脈，体温）を計ります　Let me take your blood pressure (pulse, temperature).
X線写真を撮ります　Let me take your X-ray.
日本語では「計ります」「撮ります」と使い分けますが，英語では両方 'take' でいいのです．
血液（尿）検査をします　Let me do a blood (urine) test.
'do' の後には検査の名前か種類がきます．
'Let me～' という表現と 'do,' 'take' という動詞だけを頭に入れておけば，通常の検査の場面ではほとんど困りません．
（なお，Let me run some tests. というように 'run' も使われることがあります）

『意外に通じるこの一声』

ちょっと一緒に足を踏ん張って欲しいなというとき，意外と有効なのが「一声」．こんなフレーズを覚えておくと，余分な言葉は要りません．試してみて！

- 患者さんと息を合わせる掛け声は 'One-two-three' で通じます．'Up we go!' という威勢のいいのもありました．
- もうすこしそのまま，という一瞬には 'Hold on!'．もうちょっと 'Hang on!'
- よくやったね，の気持ちは 'Good job, John!' 'Good work, Mrs. Smith' のように名前を呼ぶとしっかり伝わるはず．

このごろがんばってリハビリしているわねと声を掛けたら，You see?（わかるかい？）とうれしそうににっこり．Yes, indeed.（もちろんよ）と答えたら，がぜん元気が出たようで，That's the spirit!（そうこなくっちゃ）ですって．立場逆転．

リハビリ中の患者さんは得意になって，できるようになったことを次々見せてくれます．そんなときはこちらも素直に驚いて見せることが肝心．「すごい！」の気持ちを表すいろいろな表現には次のようなものがあります．

'Wow!' 'Lovely!' 'Super!' 'Excellent!' 'Great!' 'Fabulous!' 'No way!'.

けれど，調子に乗りすぎは禁物．もうそのくらいにした方がいいんじゃないと 'Leave it at that.'（ほどほどにしましょうね）と，適当なところでやめてもらうことも大事です．'Ouch!'（しまった．痛い！）という前に．

Unit 9 | Let's start your treatment.
処置をしましょう

Talk 9

Ns : Can I give you an intravenous drip injection now?
　　（今から点滴を始めてもよろしいですか）

Pt : Yes, please.　What kind of intravenous drip injection is it?
　　（はい，どうぞ．何の点滴ですか）

Ns : It's an antibiotic.
　　（抗生物質の点滴です）

Pt : How long will it take?
　　（どのくらい時間がかかるのでしょうか）

Ns : We are going to give you 100 ml.　It will take about 30 minutes. You'd better go to the toilet before we start.
　　（100 mlを点滴します．約30分かかります．始める前にトイレへ行かれた方がいいですよ）

Pt : I already went.
　　（済ませました）

Ns : Push the call button if you feel very hot.
　　（もしも，かっと熱い感じがしたら，ナースコールを押してください）

◘　'I'll 〜' と 'I'm going to 〜'　◘

いろいろな処置をするとき，「〜をします」は普通 'I'm going to 〜' を使います．
「点滴をします」は 'I'm going to give you an intravenous drip injection.' です．
しかし，理由が後にくる場合は，'I'll 〜' を使うことが多いです．
「痛みを和らげるために点滴をします」は 'I'll give you an intravenous drip injection to relieve the pain' となります．

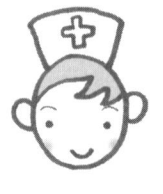

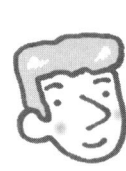

Lesson 9

A. 処置のための表現

①点滴をします	I'm going to give you an intravenous drip injection.
②傷の消毒をします	I'll disinfect the wound.
③止血します	I'll stop the bleeding.
④切開します	I'll make an incision.
⑤膿を出します	I'll press out the pus.
⑥傷のまわりの毛を剃ります	I'm going to shave away the hair around the wound.
⑦〜に温湿布をします	I'll put a hot compress on your 〜
⑧浣腸をします	I'm going to give you an enema.
⑨指で便をだします	I'll try to remove the stool with my fingers.
⑩注射をします	I'll give you an injection.　（I'll give you a shot.）
⑪少しチクっとしますよ	This may hurt a little.
⑫終わりそうになったらナースコールで呼んでください	Please push the call button, when it is almost finished.

B. 姿勢・体位・動作を示す表現

⑬立ち上がってください	Stand up.
⑭真っ直ぐに立ってください	Stand up straight.
⑮（立った状態から）座ってください	Sit down.
⑯背筋を伸ばして座ってください	Sit up straight.
⑰深く座ってください	Sit back.
⑱（寝た状態から）起き上がってください	Sit up.
⑲ベッドに横になってください	Lie down on the bed.
⑳ベッドに座ってください	Sit on the bed.
㉑右を下にして横になってください	Lie on your right side.
㉒仰向けになってください	Lie on your back.
㉓腹ばいになってください	Lie on your stomach.
㉔仰向きに寝て，膝を立ててください	Lie on your back and bend your knees.
㉕反対側を向いてください	Turn over.
㉖右をむいてください	Turn to the right.

㉗あごを引いてください　　　　　Draw in your chin.
㉘胸を張ってください　　　　　　Throw out your chest.
㉙前へ腕を伸ばしてください　　　Stretch out your arms forward.
㉚足を揃えてください　　　　　　Stand with your legs together.
㉛足を伸ばしてください　　　　　Stretch out your legs.
㉜足は内股にしてください．　　　Point your toes inward.
㉝（座位で）足元を引いてください　　Draw in your legs.

㉞私の手を握ってください　　　　Hold my hand.
㉟手をだしてください　　　　　　May I have your hand?
㊱力を入れてください（筋肉を緊張させる）　Tighten your muscles.
㊲力をぬいてください　　　　　　Please relax.

㊳息を吸って吐いてください　　　Breathe in and out.
㊴大きく息を吸ってください　　　Breathe in deeply.
㊵息を止めてください　　　　　　Hold your breath.
㊶口を大きくあけてください　　　Open your mouth wide.
㊷アーと言ってください　　　　　Say "a-a-ah."

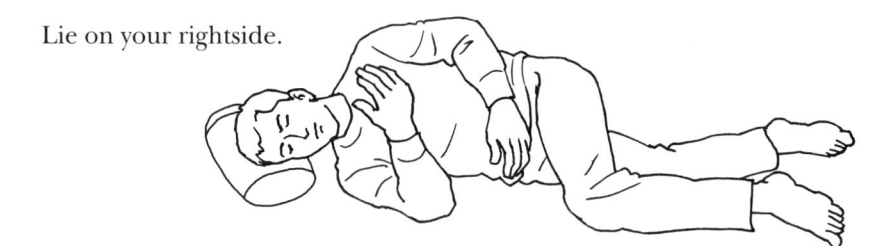

Lie on your rightside.

Lie on your back and bend your knees.

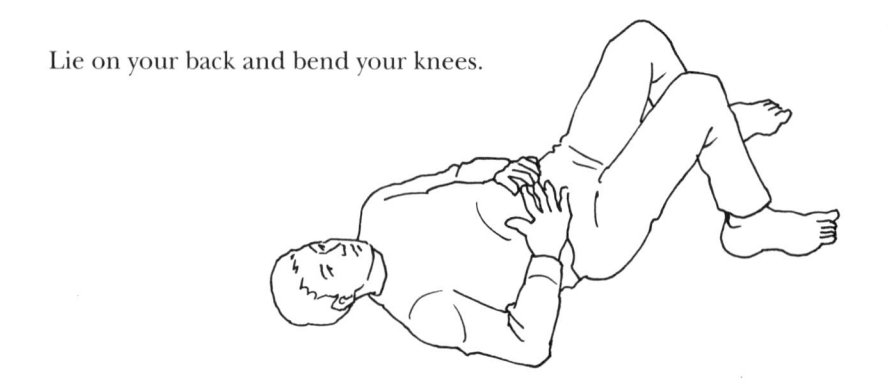

Exercise 9

Listen to the CD and fill in the blanks.
(CDを聞いて，下線部分をうめなさい)

1. I have to disinfect the _____.
   (傷の消毒をしなければなりません)
2. I'll wrap this _____ around your arm.
   (腕に包帯をします)
3. You will receive an _____ _____ twice a day.
   (1日に2回静脈注射をします)
4. Please hold this _____ firmly in place.
   (ガーゼをしっかり押さえていてください)
5. _____ out your right _____.
   (右腕を伸ばしてください)
6. _____ _____ your side and bend your knees to your chest.
   (横になって膝を胸のほうにまげてください)
7. Lie on your _____ on the examination couch.
   (診察台の上に腹ばいになってください)
8. The _____ did not work.
   (浣腸は効果がなかったです)
9. Is it going to _____?
   (痛いですか)
10. Why are you _____ around the wound?
    (どうして傷の回りの毛を剃るのですか)

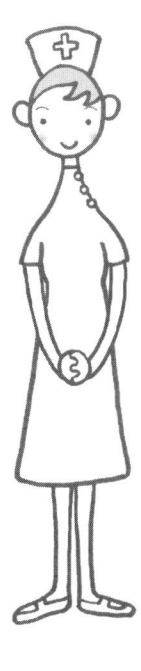

知っておきたい用語

1) 処置用語

静脈注射	intravénous injéction	皮下注射	subcutáneous injéction
皮内注射	intradérmal injéction	筋肉注射	intramúscular injéction
点滴	intravénous drip injection	消毒	disinféction
消毒液	disinféctant medicátion	止血	stópping the bléeding
切開	incísion	膿	pus
剃毛	sháving	湿布	compréss
浣腸	énema	摘便	mánual remóval of fécal impáction
吸入	inhalátion	挿管	intubátion
カニューレ挿入	cannulátion	吸引	súction
麻酔	anesthésia	人工呼吸	artifícial respirátion
輸血	blood transfúsion	切開（法）	incísion
縫合	súture	帝王切開	Caesárean séction
カテーテル法	catheterizátion	透析	diálysis

2) 医療用具

診察台	examinátion cóuch		
注射器	injéctor, syrínge	針	néedle
ピンセット	twéezers	メス	scálpel
カテーテル	cátheter	浣腸器	énema
吸入器	inháler	舌圧子	tóngue depréssor
綿棒	cótton swab	包帯	bándage
ガーゼ	gauze（dressing）	ばんそうこう	plástic bándage
テープ	adhésive tape	三角巾	cravát
副木	splínter	ギプス	cast
コルセット	córset	サポーター	suppórter
担架	strétcher	車椅子	whéelchair
松葉杖	crutch	歩行器	wálker

★☆★☆★☆★☆★☆★☆　人体各部の名称（2）　★☆★☆★☆★☆★☆★☆★

処置をするときなど体の主な部位を知っていると便利です．ここでは体の外部の用語をまとめました．体の内部についてはUnit 7を見てください．

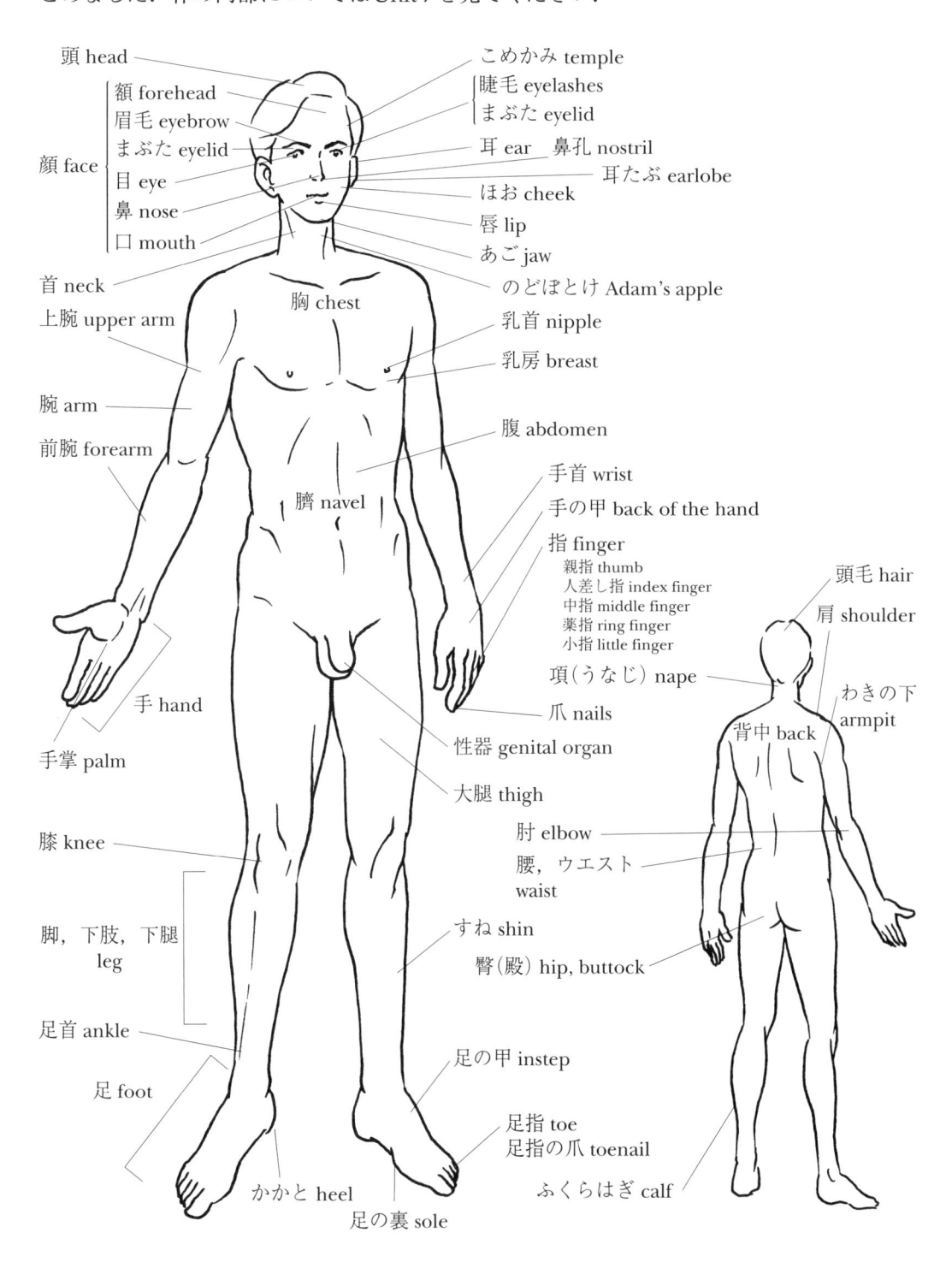

頭 head
顔 face
　額 forehead
　眉毛 eyebrow
　まぶた eyelid
　目 eye
　鼻 nose
　口 mouth
こめかみ temple
睫毛 eyelashes
まぶた eyelid
耳 ear　鼻孔 nostril
耳たぶ earlobe
ほお cheek
唇 lip
あご jaw
首 neck
のどぼとけ Adam's apple
胸 chest
乳首 nipple
乳房 breast
上腕 upper arm
腕 arm
前腕 forearm
腹 abdomen
臍 navel
手首 wrist
手の甲 back of the hand
指 finger
　親指 thumb
　人差し指 index finger
　中指 middle finger
　薬指 ring finger
　小指 little finger
手 hand
手掌 palm
爪 nails
性器 genital organ
大腿 thigh
肘 elbow
腰，ウエスト waist
膝 knee
脚，下肢，下腿 leg
すね shin
臀（殿）hip, buttock
足首 ankle
足 foot
足の甲 instep
足指 toe
足指の爪 toenail
かかと heel
足の裏 sole
ふくらはぎ calf

頭毛 hair
肩 shoulder
項（うなじ）nape
わきの下 armpit
背中 back

Unit 10

Please take this medicine.
薬を飲んでください

Talk 10

Ns : This is the painkiller. I'll give you 5 tablets all together.
　　（痛み止めです．5錠お渡ししておきます）

Pt : Five tablets at one time?
　　（1回5錠ですか）

Ns : No! Take only one tablet at a time when you are in pain.
　　（いいえ，1回1錠，痛いときにご自分で飲んでください）

Pt : Can I take one more tablet, if it doesn't work?
　　（痛みが取れなければもう1錠のんでもいいですか）

Ns : Push the call button, and ask a nurse first.
　　（そのときは，ナースコールでまずナースに知らせてください）

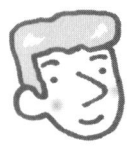

◆　与薬方法の表現　◆

薬を「～する」という動詞は，薬の形状によって違ってきます．

飲む	take（tablet, pill, capsule, powder, syrup）
塗る	apply（ointment, cream, liniment）
塗りこむ	rub（ointment）
使う	use（gargle, inhaler, mouthwash）
なめる	suck on（troche）
点眼する	put in（eye drops）
する	give you（a suppository, injection）
挿入する	insert（a suppository）

Lesson 10

Nurse

①お薬のアレルギーはありますか　Do you have any drug allergy?

②お薬を水でのんでください　　　Please take this medicine with water.

③お薬はお茶でのまないでください　Please do not take the medicine with tea.

④毎食後30分以内に飲んでください

　　　　　　　　　　　　　　Take this medicine within 30 minutes after each meal.

⑤心臓がどきどきするようなら，連絡してください

　　　　　　　　　　　　　　If your heart beats quickly, please let us know.

⑥これは坐薬です．肛門から挿入します

　　　　　　　　　　　　　　This is a suppository.　Insert it into the anus.

⑦処方せんを確かめましょう　　Let's check the prescription.

⑧お薬を飲んで具合が悪くなったら教えてください

　　　　　　　　　　　　　　Please let us know if you do not feel well after taking this medicine.

⑨このお薬を飲んだとき何か具合の悪いことがありましたか

　　　　　　　　　　　　　　Did you have any side effect when you took this medicine?

Patient

⑩このお薬は何のお薬ですか　　What's this medicine good for?

⑪このお薬は1日何回飲めばよいのでしょうか

　　　　　　　　　　　　　　How many times should I take this medicine a day?

⑫このお薬は1回に何錠のめばよいのでしょうか

　　　　　　　　　　　　　　How many tablets should I take at one time?

⑬このお薬を飲むとかゆくなります　I feel itchy after taking this medicine.

⑭今日のお薬は変わったのですか　Have you changed my medicine today?

⑮身体が熱く感じますが，薬のせいでしょうか

　　　　　　　　　　　　　　I feel hot. Is this a side effect of my medicine?

Exercise 10

Listen to the CD and fill in the blanks.
（CDを聞いて，下線部分をうめなさい）

1. You may get a little feverish when you take this _____.
   （この鎮痛剤を飲むと少し熱が出るかもしれません）
2. When you are in pain, take three _____ at one time.
   （1回3錠，痛いときにご自分で飲んでください）
3. Take one tablet three times a day _____ _____ _____.
   （1日3回毎食後1錠ずつのんでください）
4. You should take _____ as scheduled.
   （抗生物質を時間どおりに飲まなければいけませんよ）
5. This _____ _____ doesn't work well.
   （この睡眠薬はあまり効きません）
6. You can stop taking this _____, if you feel good.
   （気分がよくなったらこの薬は飲まなくていいです）
7. Take two _____ as soon as you get up in the morning.
   （朝起きたらすぐに丸薬2錠を飲んでください）
8. Please put in _____ _____ three times a day.
   （1日3回目薬をさしてください）
9. Please apply this _____ yourself.
   （ご自分でこの軟膏を塗ってください）
10. You have to insert the _____ into your anus.
    （肛門から坐薬を入れてください）

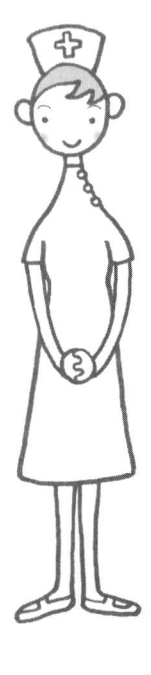

知っておきたい用語

1) 薬の服用

飲む回数や時間

1日1回	once a day
1日2回	twice a day
食前に	before a meal (before meals)
食後に	after a meal (after meals)
食間に	between meals
食後30分後に	thirty minutes after a meal
入眠前に	at bedtime
6時間ごとに	every six hours
1日1回起床時	once a day at the time of rising
1日3回毎食後	three times a day after each meal
痛みのあるときに	anytime when you are in pain, as necessary for pain
せきの出るときに	as necessary for cough
必要時に	as needed

薬の分量

1/2錠	a half tablet, half a tablet
小さじ1杯分	a spoonful of
1目盛り	one part (unit) measure
1アンプル	one ampule
2カプセル	two capsules

2) 薬の種類――薬効別

睡眠薬	sléeping pill	精神安定剤	tránquilizer
鎮静剤	sédative	麻酔薬	anesthétic
抗生物質	antibiótic	抗菌剤	antimicróbial agent
鎮痛剤	páinkiller	解熱剤	antifébrile
消炎剤	antiphlogístic	風邪薬	cold médicine
咳止め	cough médicine	咳止めシロップ	lózenge
うがい薬	gárgle, móuthwash	消毒薬	disinféctant
降圧薬	antihyperténsive ágent	昇圧薬	vasopréssor
利尿薬	diurétic	強心薬	cardiotónic

胃薬	stómach médicine	消化薬	digéstive médicine
制酸薬	antácid médicine	抗潰瘍薬	antiulcerative
下剤	láxative	止痢剤	antidiarrhéa
利胆剤	chólagogue		
抗がん薬	anticáncer drug	免疫抑制剤	immunosuppréssant
解毒剤	ántidote		
造血剤	haematínic	止血剤	stýptic
抗糖尿病薬	antidiabétic	抗ヒスタミン剤	antihístamine
漢方薬	Chinése hérbal médicine / Kanpo		

3) 薬の種類——用法別

経口薬（内用薬）

錠剤	táblet	カプセル	cápsule
丸薬	pill	顆粒	gránule
散剤	pówder	水薬	líquid
舌下薬	sublíngual médicine		

外用薬

軟膏，塗布薬	óintment	はり薬，湿布薬	pláster
坐薬	suppósitory		
吸入薬	inhálant		
点眼薬	eye drops		
点鼻薬	nose drops		

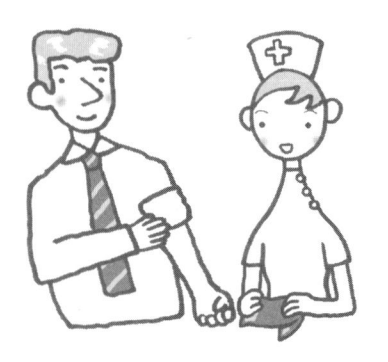

**************応用フレーズ**************

お薬を飲んで10分ぐらいで眠くなりますよ
       You'll feel sleepy in about 10 minutes after taking this medicine.
このお薬はあまりききませんのでお薬を変えてもらえませんか
       This medicine doesn't work well.　Will you change my medicine?
急にこんなぶつぶつが出て痒くなりました．これはお薬の影響ですか
   I suddenly developed a rashe and feel itchy.　Is this a side effect of the medicine?

『安心の医療』

　単身来日した女性が，子供ができたかも，と産婦人科を受診しました．妊娠は初めてで，家族からも離れています．日本語もあまりわからず，お金もどのくらいかかるかわかりません．
　心配だらけで街の医師の診察を受けに行ったところ，幸運にも言葉の通じる医師に出会い，納得のいく説明をしてもらえました．質問も正しく理解してくれました．最後に，あなたも赤ちゃんも大丈夫ですよ，と言われてすっかり安心したそうです．
　「でも，今回はラッキーだったけど，言葉の通じないときも多いわよね．そういうとき妙に調子よく『大丈夫！』とか言われても，かえって心配になっちゃう…」と彼女は言います．
　『…どき！』
　逃げ腰の説明は丸見えなのね．やっぱり安請け合いはダメダメ．

　「そういう時は，書いてもらうようにしているの，キーワードだけでもいいのよ」
　『そうか！』
　そうすれば，その場でわからないことでも，後で調べることができるわけです．詳しい友達に尋ねることもできるでしょう．患者さんも工夫してるんだなあ！
　「はじめての子供を授かったのです．自分の身体のことだけではないのですから，確信を持てるまで納得しておきたいの…」と，彼女は楽しそうな様子です．
　外国人が安心して子どもを産めることを，日本人として少し誇らしく感じました．

Unit 11　I'm sure the results will be good.
きっといい結果になりますよ

Talk 11

Ns : It will be over in a moment.
　　（もうすぐ終わりますからね）

Pt : How long will it take?　I feel numbness around my arm.
　　（あとどのくらいですか　腕がしびれてきました）

Ns : You'll feel better soon.
　　（すぐ楽になりますよ）

Pt : Will it be over soon?
　　（もう終わりますか）

Ns : Just a little bit more.　I'm sure the results will be good.
　　（あとひとふんばりです．きっといい結果になりますよ）

『心のコミュニケーション』

　言葉そのものによるコミュニケーション（verbal communication）だけでなく，声の調子，イントネーション，顔の表情，しぐさ等の，言葉以外によるコミュニケーション（non-verbal communication）も大切です．患者さんを理解しようとする気持ちがあれば，non-verbal communication で自然に外国の方とも気持ちをうまく伝え合えます．英語がほとんどできなくても心と心のコミュニケーションはできるといっても過言ではないかもしれません．

　でも，英語のちょっとした言い回しを知っているだけで，外国からの患者さんとのコミュニケーションが一層深まることは言うまでもありません．気に入ったものだけでいいですから，頭の中に入れておきましょう．「気軽に声をかけましょう」の会話例も参考にしてください．

　non-verbal communication の1つであるジェスチャーで，注意しないといけない点があります．「こちらへいらっしゃい」と日本では手招きするジェスチャーがありますが，欧米ではこのジェスチャーは「あちらへ行きなさい」という逆の意味になります．国によって随分違うので，気をつけましょう．

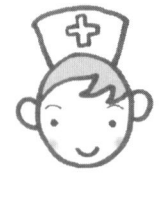

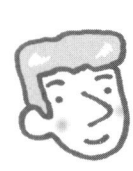

Lesson 11

1) 励まし，気持ちを楽にする表現

①大丈夫ですよ	It will be all right. /It will be fine.
	Everything will go well.
②すぐ，よくなりますよ	You will be fine soon.
③心配しないでください	Don't worry.
④あきらめないでください	Don't give up.
⑤楽にしてください	Try to relax.
⑥あと5分で終わりますからね	You'll be finished in five minutes.
⑦これで全部済みましたよ	It's all over.
⑧できますとも	Sure, you can.
⑨がんばって	Good luck!
⑩わたしの手を握っていてください	Hold my hand.
⑪そばについていますからね	I'll stay with you.
⑫私がお手伝いします	I'll help you.
⑬それをきいて私もうれしいです	I'm pleased to hear that.
⑭次のステップに挑戦ですね	Now let's try the next step.
⑮大変でしたね．よくがんばりました	Well done. Thank you.
⑯きっとうまくいきますよ（手術など）	I'm sure it will be successful.
⑰いい考えかも知れませんよ．やってみましょう	It might be a good idea. Let's try.

2) 制止の表現

⑱そのままで！この位置で動かないで下さい	Please hold still. Please don't move.
⑲急に動いてはだめです．危険ですよ	Don't move suddenly. It's dangerous.
⑳まだ立ち上がらないで下さい	Please don't stand up.
㉑待って．もうちょっとこのままで	Wait. Please hold still for a moment.
㉒ここを離れないで下さい	Stay where you are.
㉓そこを触らないで下さい	Don't touch there.
㉔今は入らないで下さい．処置中です	Don't come in now. We're giving treatment.
㉕ゆっくりでいいですよ．あわててはだめです	Please do it slowly. Calm yourself.
㉖まだ，飲みこんではだめです	Don't swallow it down.
㉗すみませんがまだ食べずにいて下さい	Excuse me, but please don't eat yet.

◆　気軽に声をかけましょう　◆

その1

Ns：　今日はお加減いかがですか　　　How are you feeling today?
　　　　　　　　　　　　　　　　　　How are you today?
　　　　　　　　　　　　　　　　　　How are you doing?
　　　　　　　　　　　　　　　　　　How are things going?

Pt1：とてもいいです　　　　　　　　Fine
　　　最高です　　　　　　　　　　　Never better
　　　なかなかいいです　　　　　　　Pretty good
　　　悪くはありません　　　　　　　Not bad, thank you.

Ns：　それはよかった！　　　　　　　Good!

Pt2：　あまりよくありません　　　　　Not so good

Ns：　まあ，どうされましたか　　　　What's the problem?

Pt3：　昨日よりはいいです．まあまあです
　　　　　　　　　　　　　　　　　　I'm feeling better than yesterday. So so.

Ns：　よかったですね　　　　　　　　That's OK.

Pt4：　ひどい状態です　　　　　　　　Terrible.

Ns：　それは，いけませんね．安静にしていてください
　　　　　　　　　　　　　　　　　　Too bad! You must stay in bed.

Pt5：　どう見えます　　　　　　　　　How do I look?

Ns：　すこし寝不足ぎみのようにみえますが
　　　　　　　　　　　　　　　　　　You don't seem to have slept well.

その2

Ns：　よく眠れましたか　　　　　　　Have you been sleeping well?

Pt1：　ええ，朝までぐっすり寝ました
　　　　　　　　　　　　　　　　　　Yes, I have been sleeping soundly till morning.

Pt2：　眠りが浅いみたいです．なんどか目が覚めました
　　　　　　　　　　　　　　　　　　I have been sleeping badly. I woke up many times.

Pt3：　薬のおかげで，夢も見ないで眠っていました
　　　　　　　　　　　　　　　　　　I have been sleeping without a dream owing to the medicine.

Pt4：　トイレが近くて困ります　　　　I have to wake up to go to the toilet many times.

Pt5：　3時に起きました　　　　　　　I woke up at 3 o'clock.

Pt6：　寝苦しくて朝までが長かったです
　　　　　　　　　　　　　　　　　　I slept very badly and it was a long night for me.

Exercise 11

Listen to the CD and fill in the blanks.
（CDを聞いて，下線部分をうめなさい）

1. It will be _____ in three minutes.
   （あと3分で終わりますからね）
2. I'm _____ you'll be _____ soon.
   （必ずすぐによくなりますよ）
3. Don't _____ _____. I'll always stay with you.
   （あきらめないで．いつもそばにいますから）
4. Please _____ _____.
   （動かないで）
5. _____ ___ open the window?
   （窓を開けましょうか）
6. You shouldn't _____ ___ _____ tonight.
   （今夜はお風呂に入ってはいけません）
7. _____ _____ _____ something when you feel better.
   （気分がよくなったら食べてください）
8. You cannot _____ here.
   （ここで煙草をすってはいけません）
9. Please _____ _____ _____, when you go out.
   （院外へ出るときはナースにお知らせください）
10. It's past _____. I will turn off the light.
    （消灯時間は過ぎましたので，電気を消しますよ）

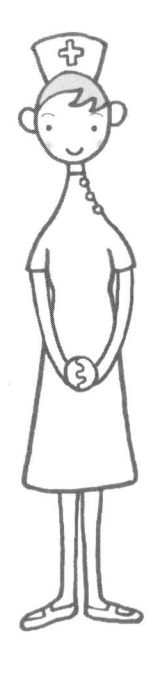

*************** 応用フレーズ ***************

（ベッドで快適に）

寒くないですか	Aren't you cold?
毛布を1枚足しておきますね	I'll cover you with one more blanket.
毛布を持ってきましょうか	Shall I bring a blanket?
枕を替えてみましょうか	Shall I change the pillow?
シーツを交換しましょうか	Shall I change your sheets?
少し姿勢を変えてみましょう．こうするとどうですか	Let's change your position. How about it?
今日はどのパジャマにしますか	Which pajamas are you going to wear?
窓を閉めましょうか	Shall I close the window?

（お風呂）

久しぶりにお風呂にでもはいったらいかがですか	Why don't you try taking a bath after a long absence?
まだ，お風呂に入るのは難しいですよ	You cannot take a bath now.
ここを右にひねると，カランからお湯が出ます	Turn here clockwise. Hot water will come out from a faucet.
温度を確認してください	See how hot it is.
温度の調整はこのダイヤルです	You can control the temperature with this dial.
髪を洗いましょうか．シャンプーは決まったものをお使いですか	Shall I shampoo your hair? Do you have your favorite shampoo?
まだ，タオルの替えがありますか	Are there other clean towels?

（トイレ）

トイレに行くときは，ナースがつきそいますので，知らせてくださいね	The nurse will support you when you go to the toilet. Please let us know.
トイレに行くのが無理なら，カモードを使いましょうか	How about using a commode chair, if you cannot go to the toilet?
明日の朝，最初に排尿するときに，ナースに声をかけてください	Please call a nurse, when you go to the toilet first tomorrow morning.

〔食事〕

あまり食べていませんね	You haven't eaten very much.
食事はおいしく召し上がりましたか	Did you enjoy your dinner?
朝食をしっかり食べてください	I hope you'll have your breakfast enough.
少しでも食べてください	Please try to eat some.

〔消灯時間〕

消灯時間が過ぎましたので，テレビを消してください	The lights-out is over.　Please turn off the T.V.
寝る時間ですよ	It's time to sleep.
明かりを消しましょうか	Shall I turn off the light?
ぐっすり眠ってください	Please have a good sleep.

◆　覚えておきたい英語表現パターン　◆

患者さんに何かをしてもらわなければならないとき，患者さんに提案するとき，ナースに知らせてもらう必要があるとき，また患者さんからの同意を求める場合など，日々よく使う表現の原型を集めてみました．中学校で習った簡単な英語なのですが，実際の場面になるとなかなか口から出てこないものです．是非これだけは反射的に出るようにしておきましょう．

「～してください」Please ～動詞原形 .
「～しないでください」Please do not ～動詞原形 .
「～しないでいいです」You don't have to ～動詞原形 .
「～してみたらいかがですか？」Why don't you ～動詞原形 ?
「～させていただきたいのですが」I would like to ～動詞原形 .
「～しましょうか？」Shall I ～動詞原形 ?
「知らせてください」Please let us know.
「ナースを呼んでください」Please call a nurse.

Unit 12

Now, you can leave the hospital.
いよいよ退院ですね

Talk 12

Ns : Please pay at the cashier.
　　（会計でお支払いを済ませてください）

Pt : I've finished.　Here's the receipt.
　　（済ませました．領収書です）

Ns : Here is your medicine for 2 weeks, appointment card, and ID card.
　　（それではこれが，2週間分のお薬と，外来の予約券，そして診察券です）

Pt : Thank you.
　　（有難うございます）

Ns : Be sure to bring this ID card and health insurance card when you come to the outpatient department.
　　（外来受診の日は，この診察券と保険証を忘れずにお持ちください）

Pt : OK.
　　（はい）

Ns : Please call this number, if you wish to change the appointment.
　　（予約日の変更の場合には，ここへお電話いただけますか）

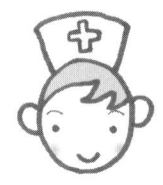

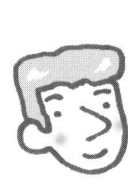

Pt : OK.
　　（わかりました）

Lesson 12

Nurse

①おめでとうございます	Congratulations!
②退院の用意はできましたか	Are you ready to leave the hospital?
③来週退院です	You can go home next week.
④薬は続けてください	Continue taking your medicine.
⑤これは自宅で飲んでいただくお薬です	Here's the medicine you have to take at home.
⑥2週間ごとに外来受診をしてください	Please come to see the doctor every 2 weeks.
⑦定期的に受診してください	Please come back regularly.
⑧最初の予約をいつにしますか	When shall I make an appointment for you?
⑨紹介状を先方の病院に渡してください	Please take this referral letter to the hospital.
⑩どなたか迎えにこられますか	Will anyone come to get you?
⑪早くよくなってください	I wish you a speedy recovery.
⑫ケースワーカーを紹介しましょうか	Would you like to be introduced to a case worker?
⑬お元気で	Take good care of yourself.

Patient

⑭退院はいつになるでしょうか	When will I be able to leave the hospital?
⑮大西医師の診察日はいつですか	What day of the week can Dr. Oonishi see me?
⑯ありがとう．いろいろお世話になりました	Thank you very much for everything.

Exercise 12

Listen to the CD and fill in the blanks.
(CDを聞いて，下線部分をうめなさい)

1. _____! You can go home tomorrow.
   (おめでとうございます．明日ご退院ですね)

2. Please come to see the doctor _____ _____ _____ after you leave the hospital.
   (退院後は2ヶ月ごとに受診してください)

3. Shall I make an _____ for you?
   (予約をおとりしましょうか)

4. Dr. Yamamoto _____ _____ you any weekday except Wednesday.
   (山本医師の診察日は水曜日以外です)

5. Please _____ at the _____ on the second floor.
   (2階の会計でお支払いをしてください)

6. When will I have to _____ _____ to see the doctor next?
   (今度いつ受診すればいいのですか)

7. Can I do without a painkiller after I _____ _____?
   (退院後は鎮痛剤を使わずにすむでしょうか)

8. Will you introduce a good home-care _____ _____ to me?
   (良い訪問看護サービスを紹介してもらえませんか)

9. What day of the _____ can my doctor-in-charge see me?
   (主治医の先生には何曜日に診ていただけるのでしょうか)

10. Thank you very much ____ _____ you have done for me.
    (いろいろお世話になりありがとうございました)

知っておきたい用語

訪問看護師	vísiting nurse
保健師	públic health nurse
助産師	mídwife
ケアマネージャー，介護支援専門員	care mánager
ホームヘルパー	home helper
かかりつけ医	fámily dóctor
一般開業医	géneral practítioner
患者を紹介してきた医師	reférring dóctor
健康保険	health insúrance
健康保険証	health insúrance card
保険料	insúrance prémiums
訪問看護サービス	home care núrsing service
保健所	públic health cénter
有料老人ホーム	private núrsing home
グループホーム	group home for sénile péople

『自己決定の重み』

　イギリス人の老紳士と，末期の癌と診断された妻の療養について相談したときのことです．医師から，妻の病気がとても進行していることや，これから先，痛みが出てきたり食事がとれなくなったり，点滴も必要になるだろう，奥さんの状態から考えるとホスピスへ入所を勧める，といったことが伝えられました．

　しかし，夫は，家へ連れて帰って療養させるというのです．二人ともかなり高齢で，二人暮らしでしたから，担当したケースワーカーは心配でした．必要になる介護の大変さについてわかっていないのではと思い，確認しましたが，医師から説明されたことについて，夫は良く理解しているようでした．

　ケースワーカーは，本当は心配だけど何か言えない事情があって無理してうちに帰ると言っているのではと考えました．そういうことは日本人の家族にはよくあることだったからです．しかし，夫はすっきりと「治療して治るのならどこでも入院するが，治らないのならば家へ帰る」と言いました．結局，介護保険の制度を活用して，訪問看護やヘルパーのサービスを受けながら，妻は自宅で亡くなったそうです．

　自分たちで最後の過ごし方を決めたのは，この夫婦にとって大きな誇りだったのではないでしょうか．その決定を権利としてまた責任として尊重したことが，この夫婦を大切にすることにつながっています．

*************** 応用フレーズ ***************

予定通りならば金曜日には退院になります．なにかお困りですか
　　　　　　　　　　You are supposed to leave here on Friday.　Do you have any problem?
来週から仕事に出ても大丈夫ですよ　　You can go to your office from next week.
地域にある制度を使うことができますよ
　　　　　　　　　　　　　　　　　　You can use the community-support system.
ヘルパーの依頼を希望されますか　　Do you want to ask for helpers?
サービスについての資料がありますよ　　Here is a brochure explaining the service.
在宅医療室に相談してみましょうか
　　　　　　　　　　　　Shall I ask the consultation room for home care nursing?
ここは救急病院なので，症状が安定したら別の病院に転院してください
　　　　　　　　　　　　　　This hospital is an emergency one.　You will be
　　　　　　　　　　　　　　moved to another hospital when you get better
1階の会計でお支払いを済ませてください
　　　　　　　　　　　　　　Please pay at the cashier on the first floor.

どんなサービスがあるか，教えてもらえますか
　　　　　　　　　　　　　　May I ask what kind of service they have?
職場には来週からは出られると言ってきたのです
　　　　　　　　　　　　　　I told my office I'll be able to return next week.

◆　次の来院の予約を取る　◆

　退院していく患者さんは，次に外来受診される時の予約をとっておく必要があります．
　日本語の「予約を取る」は英語にすると 'make a reservation' と 'make an appointment' の2種類があります．
　'make a reservation' は「空間を予約する」という意味で，飛行機の座席，ホテルの部屋，コンサートの座席等を予約する場合に使います．
　'make an appointment' は「（誰かの）時間を予約する」という意味で，取引先の社長，病院のドクター等のある時間帯（10：00〜10：30）をとってもらうときに使います．
　「次の外来の予約を取っておきましょうか？」の場合は 'Shall I make an appointment for you?' となります．予約は何でも「リザーブ」だと思っていませんか？
　一方，入院するときにベッドの予約をとる場合は「ベッドという空間」ですので，'Shall I make a reservation for you?' となります．

Unit 13 | In the outpatient department
病院外来で

Talk 13

Ns : Please come in. The doctor will see you now.
   (どうぞお入りください．ドクターが診察します)

Pt : Thank you.
   (ありがとう)

Ns : Please take off your shirt and put it into this basket.
   (シャツを脱いで，このカゴの中に入れてください)

Pt : OK.
   (はい)

Ns : Lie down facing upward on the couch.
   (診察台の上に仰向けになってください)

(After the doctor sees the patient....医師の診察後)

Ns : Please come back next Friday. And take care.
   (来週の金曜日にまたきてください．どうぞお大事に)

Pt : Thank you very much.
   (どうも有難うございました)

Ns : Please do not leave your belongings here.
   (忘れ物をしないでくださいね)

Pt : OK.
   (はい)

Ns : Please take this sheet to the cashier on the first floor.
   (この書類を持って1階の会計に行ってください)

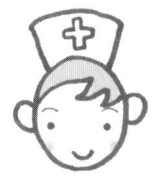

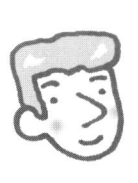

Lesson 13

Nurse

① お待たせしてすみませんでした　　I'm sorry to have kept you waiting.
② どうぞおかけください　　Please have a seat.
③ こちらは，田中先生です　　This is Dr. Tanaka.
④ 服を脱いでください　　Please take off your clothes.
⑤ 服を着てください　　Please put on your clothes.
⑥ この書類を持って放射線科に行ってください
　　Please take this paper to the X-ray department.
⑦ 放射線科は3階です　　The X-ray department is on the third floor.
⑧ X線写真を持って帰ってきてください
　　Please bring your X-ray film back with you.
⑨ 伝票を持って処置室に行ってください
　　Please take this paper and go to the treatment room.
⑩ 受付で予約をしてください　　Please make an appointment at the desk.
⑪ 入院受付で入院の手続きをしてください
　　Please fill out the necessary papers at the admission window.
⑫ 診察券をどうぞ（手渡しながら）　Here's your ID card.
⑬ 明日また来てください　　Please come back again tomorrow.
⑭ お大事に　　Take good care of yourself.

Patient

⑮ 詳しく説明してください　　Please explain in detail.
⑯ 放射線科はどこですか　　Where is the X-ray department?
⑰ 入院しなければなりませんか　　Do I have to be hospitalized?
⑱ 先生が何と言われたのかわかりませんでした
　　I didn't understand what the doctor said.
⑲ 今度はいつ来ればよいのでしょうか　　When shall I come back next?
⑳ すみませんが，お手洗いはどこですか　　Excuse me, but where is the restroom?

Exercise 13

Listen to the CD and fill in the blanks.
（CDを聞いて，下線部分をうめなさい）

1. Please _____ _____ your shoes.
   （靴をぬいでください）
2. You can put your _____ into this _____, but keep your valuables with you.
   （服はカゴの中に入れていただいて，貴重品は持っていてください）
3. Please go to the _____ for a blood test.
   （血液検査のため検査室へ行ってください）
4. The laboratory is _____ _____ the X-ray department.
   （検査室は放射線科の隣です）
5. I'll _____ _____ _____ of the second floor for you.
   （2階の地図を書きます）
6. Please go to the psychosomatic medicine _____.
   （心療内科に行ってください）
7. _____ _____ along the hall.
   （廊下に沿って真っ直ぐ行ってください）
8. _____ _____ _____ _____ on the third floor. The endoscopy department is on the left.
   （エレベーターを3階で降りてください．内視鏡検査室は左手にあります）
9. Please _____ _____ again next week.
   （来週またいらしてください）
10. Where is the _____?
    （薬局はどこですか）

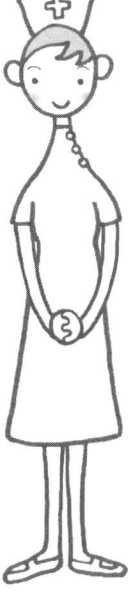

************** 応用フレーズ **************

　体調を崩して病院へ来られる患者さんにとって，目的の場所へ行くのは一苦労です．まして外国人患者さんが英文表示のない病院へ来られた時は大変なストレスになります．
　外来で，診察室から検査等に行っていただく場合，あるいは廊下で場所を聞かれた時，正確に教えてあげましょう．その場合，役立つ表現を以下にあげておきます．また病院内の各科名をあわせて覚えておくといいですよ．

どうされましたか	May I help you?
どこへ行かれるのですか	Where are you going?
まっすぐに行ってください	Go straight.
廊下に沿っていってください	Go along the hall.
右（左）に曲がってください	Turn right（left）.
右（左）手にあります	It's on the right（left）.
～の隣にあります	It's next to ～.
～と～の間にあります	It's between ～ and ～.
～の向かい側にあります	It's across from ～.
2（3）階にあります	It's on the second（third）floor.
エレベーターに乗ってください	Take the elevator.
エレベーターを6階で降りてください	Get off the elevator on the sixth floor.
階段をあがって（おりて）ください	Go up（down）the stairs.
案内図を書きます	I'll draw a map for you.
ご案内します	I'll take you there.
こちらへどうぞ	Please follow me.　Please come with me.
ここで少し待っていてください	Please wait here for a moment.
どういたしまして	You're welcome.

知っておきたい用語

1）診療科名	**Departments of medicine**	診療医	**Doctors**
内科	intérnal médicine	内科医	ínternist
循環器科	cardiólogy	循環器専門医	cardiólogist
呼吸器科	pulmonólogy	呼吸器専門医	pulmonólogist
内分泌科	endocrinólogy	内分泌専門医	endocrinólogist
消化器科	gastroenterólogy	消化器専門医	gastroenterólogist
心療内科	psychosomátic médicine	心療内科専門医	psychosomáticist
外科	súrgery	外科医	súrgeon
整形外科	orthopédics	整形外科医	orthopédist
脳神経外科	neurosúrgery	脳神経外科医	neurosúrgeon
形成外科	plástic súrgery	形成外科医	plástic súrgeon
産科	obstétrics	産科医	obstetrícian
婦人科	gynecólogy	婦人科医	gynecólogist
小児科	pediátrics	小児科医	pediatrícian
精神科	psychíatry	精神科医	psychíatrist
神経科	neurólogy	神経科医	neurólogist
泌尿器科	urólogy	泌尿器科医	urólogist
皮膚科	dermatólogy	皮膚科医	dermatólogist
放射線科	radiólogy	放射線医	radiólogist
麻酔科	anesthesiólogy	麻酔医	anesthesiólogist
耳鼻咽喉科	otorhinolaryngólogy	耳鼻咽喉科医	otorhinolaryngólogist
	ENT（ear, nose, throat）		ENT doctor
眼科	ophthalmólogy	眼科医	ophthalmólogist
			eye dóctor
歯科	déntistry	歯科医	déntist

2）病院施設名	**Facilities**		
総合受付	géneral recéption	ロビー	lóbby
新患受付	registrátion	入院受付	admíssion wíndow
外来窓口	óutpatient wíndow	3番窓口	Wíndow（Counter）No. 3
	óutpatient counter	会計窓口	cashíer
外来	óutpatient depártment	待合室	wáiting room（area）

| 診察室 | consultátion room | 処置室 | tréatment room |

放射線科	radiógraphy depártment
リハビリテーション室	rehabilitátion cénter
検査室	láboratory
採血室	blood lab
生理機能検査室	physiológical lab depártment
内視鏡検査室	endóscopy depártment
薬局	phármacy

食堂	cafetéria	喫茶室	tea room
エレベーター	élevator	廊下	hall
トイレ	lávatory, tóilet, restroom	公衆電話	públic phone, páy phone
売店	drúgstore	花屋	flórist
タクシー乗り場	táxi stand	非常口	emérgency éxit

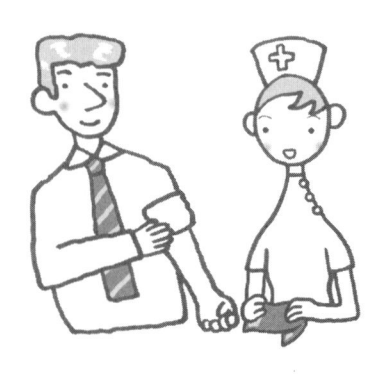

Floor Information

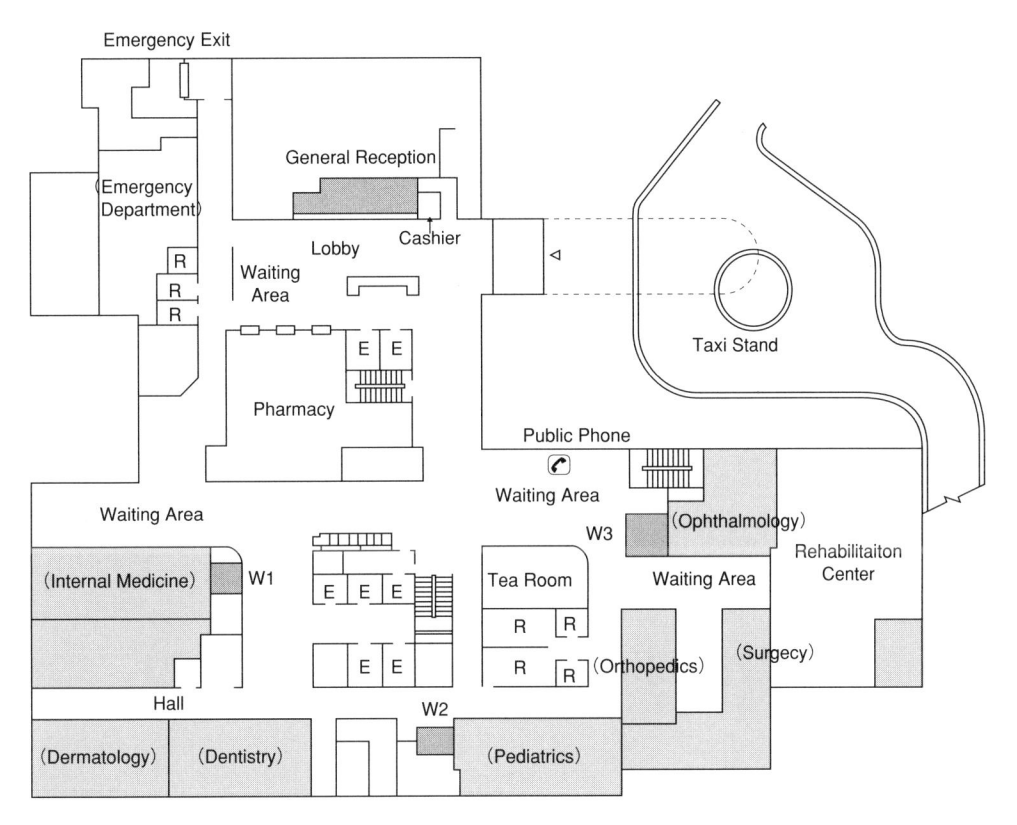

- Emergency Exit
- (Emergency Department)
- General Reception
- Cashier
- Lobby
- Waiting Area
- Pharmacy
- Taxi Stand
- Public Phone
- Waiting Area
- W3
- (Ophthalmology)
- Rehabilitaiton Center
- Waiting Area
- (Internal Medicine) W1
- Tea Room
- (Orthopedics)
- (Surgecy)
- Hall
- W2
- (Dermatology)
- (Dentistry)
- (Pediatrics)

E: Elevator
R: Rest room
W1: Window No1

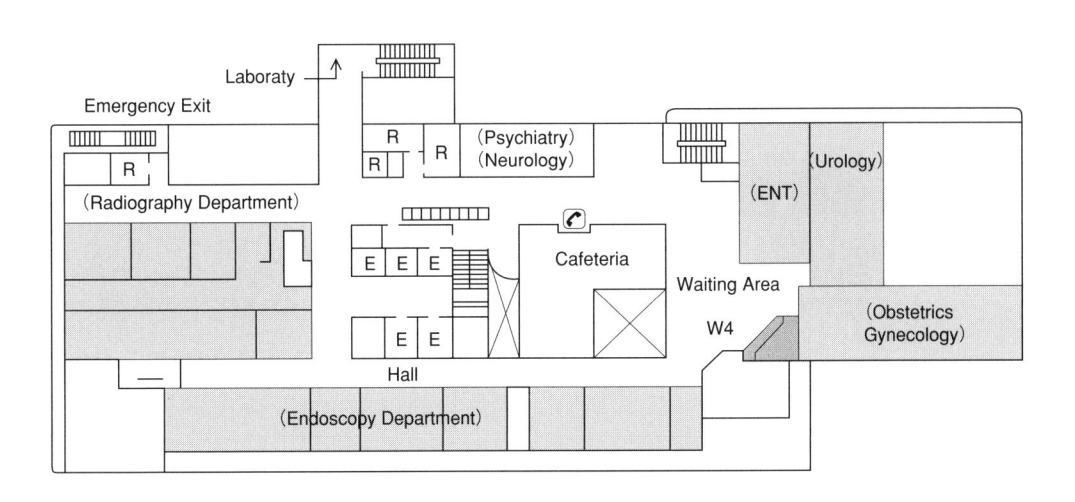

- Laboraty
- Emergency Exit
- (Psychiatry)
- (Neurology)
- (Urology)
- (ENT)
- (Radiography Department)
- Cafeteria
- Waiting Area
- W4
- (Obstetrics Gynecology)
- Hall
- (Endoscopy Department)

（神戸市立西市民病院案内図をもとに作成）

Unit 14　At the clinic
診療所で

Talk 14

Ns : Good morning.　May I help you?
（おはようございます．どうされましたか）

Pt : I have a severe headache, so I'd like to see a doctor.
（頭痛がひどいので一度診ていただきたいのです）

Ns : Do you have any health insurance card?
（健康保険証はお持ちですか）

Pt : Here's my insurance card.
（はい．これです）

Ns : Please have a seat and wait for a moment.
（かけて少しお待ちください）

(After the doctor sees the patient)（医師診察後）

Ns : Here's your medicine.　Take two tablets before each meal.　Three times a day.
（お薬をどうぞ．食事の前に2錠飲んでください．1日3回です）

Pt : OK.
（わかりました）

Clerk : Today's fee is 1,500 yen.
（本日は1,500円お支払いください）

Pt : Here you are.
（はい，どうぞ）

Clerk : Please come back next week.
（来週もう一度来てください）

Pt : Thank you very much.
（ありがとうございました）

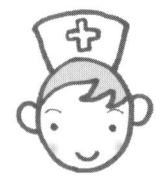

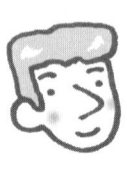

Lesson 14

①電話番号を教えてください　　　　　May I have your telephone number please?
②お名前のつづりを教えてください　　Will you spell out your name?
③ここにご住所を書いてもらえますか　Will you write your address here?
④この書類にお名前とお電話番号を書き込んで下さい
　　　　　　　　　　　　　　　Please write your name and telephone number on this form.
⑤前にも受診されたことがありますか　Have you ever been to this clinic before?

⑥これがあなたの診察券です　　　　　Here's your ID card.
⑦当院に来られる時はこの診察券をお持ちください
　　　　　　　　　　　　　　　Please bring this ID card when you come to this clinic.
⑧その月最初の受診日に保険証を持ってきてください
　　　　　　　　　　　　　　　Please bring your health insurance card on your first visit every month.
⑨何かありましたら，お電話をください　　Please call us if you have any problem.
⑩精密検査のためにB病院へ行ってください
　　　　　　　　　　　　　　　Please go to the B Hospital for a detailed examination.

⑪もしもし，学園クリニックです（電話で）　Hello. Gakuen Clinic. May I help you?
⑫トイレはむこうです　　　　　　　　The restroom is over there.
⑬子供さんをあずかりましょう　　　　I'll take care of your child.
⑭次の予約をおとりしましょう　　　　I'd like to make an appointment for you.
⑮お大事に　　　　　　　　　　　　Take care.
⑯おつりです　　　　　　　　　　　Here is your change.

（検査・処置の場面，薬の説明等についてはそれぞれのUnitを見てください）

Exercise 14

Listen to the CD and fill in the blanks.
（CDを聞いて，下線部分をうめなさい）

1. Could you please spell out your _____?
   （あなたの名字のスペルを教えていただけますか）
2. When did you last come to this _____?
   （前にいつこのクリニックに来られましたか）
3. Your telephone number is _____. Is that right?
   （お電話番号は　　　　ですね？）
4. Today's _____ is _____ yen.
   （本日の治療費は　　　円です）
5. Please come back _____ _____.
   （来月また来てください）
6. I was born in _____.
   （　　　年生まれです）
7. Do I have to _____ _____ this form myself?
   （この書類は自分で書き込まなければなりませんか）
8. Where is the _____?
   （トイレはどこですか）
9. Where do I have to go for a _____ _____?
   （精密検査のためにどこへ行かなければいけないのでしょうか）
10. I'd like to _____ _____ _____ for next Wednesday.
    （来週水曜日に予約を取っていただきたいのですが）

知っておきたい用語			
名字（姓）	súrname	名前	fírst name
年齢	age	住所	addréss
性別	sex	生誕地	bírthplace
国籍	nationálity	職業	occupátion

緊急時連絡先	emérgency cóntact
（緊急のときは〜に連絡してください　In an emergency, contact〜）	
保険証の種類	type of insúrance
保険証番号	pólicy númber
扶養家族	depéndent

『つり銭の渡し方』

　これにはお国振りがあり，日本とは欧米では違うので注意しなければなりません．例えば，日本は1,500円の料金の場合10,000円札を出されると，即座に引き算をして8,500円を返却します．一方，欧米では1,500円に足し算をしていきます．

　「1,500円」（'one thousand five hundred yen'）
　（500円玉を足して）「2,000円」（'two thousand yen'）
　（1,000円札を足して）「3,000円」（'three thousand yen'）
　（1,000円札を足して）「4,000円」（'four thousand yen'）
　（1,000円札を足して）「5,000円」（'five thousand yen'）
　（5,000円札を足して）「10,000円」（'ten thousand yen'）
　というようにして返していきます．

************** 応用フレーズ **************

健康保険証をお持ちでないと全額負担になってしまいます
　　　　　　　　　　　If you don't have health insurance card, you must pay the full fee.

電話での相談も料金をいただく場合があります
　　　　　　　　　　　　　You may be charged for consultation over the telephone.

B病院へこの紹介状を持って行ってください
　　　　　　　　　　　　Please bring this referral letter with you to B Hospital.

『数字が読めますか？』

＜金額の読み方＞

　診療費の支払いの場合，正確に金額を伝えなければなりません．単位を間違えたりすると大変です．1,500 yen は 'one thousand and five hundred yen' と読みます．全額自己負担などの場合，高額になることもありますので，数字の読み方を復習しておきましょう．

　年齢や医療費の場合に出てくる簡単な数の例をあげます．

15	fifteen
23	twenty-three
150	one hundred and fifty
3,700	three thousand and seven hundred
26,000	twenty-six thousand
35,940	thirty-five thousand, nine hundred and forty

＜電話番号の読み方＞

　電話番号は数字を1つずつ読みます．例えば07-776-3385 'zero seven, seven seven six, three three eight five' となります．なお数字の0は 'zero' または 'oh' と読む場合もあります．次の番号を読んでみましょう．

　　　　04-5982-3490
　　　　063-980-3511
　　　　07-793-0028
　　　　08-363-9284

＜年号＞

　生年月日は保険証があれば，書いてありますが，ない場合は尋ねなければなりません．普通の数字の読み方（上の金額の場合など）とは違いますので注意してください．西暦の年号の読み方を復習しておきましょう．

　　　　1936（nineteen thirty-six）
　　　　1957（nineteen fifty-seven）
　　　　1970（nineteen seventy）
　　　　2002（two thousand two）

Appendix

Children's world, children's words
子供の世界，子供のことば

①えらかったね	You were very good.
	Good job!
②つよい子だったね	You did fine.
③どうしてこんなにつよい子だったのでしょう！	How could you be so brave!
④おりこうさんだったわね	You were very good.
⑤大丈夫，痛くないわよ	Don't worry. It's not going to hurt.
⑥ちょっと目をつぶっていてね	Please keep your eyes shut for a moment.
⑦終わったよ	I'm all done.
⑧いい子にしていてね	Be a good boy.
⑨お行儀よくしていてね	Behave yourself.
⑩静かにしていてね	Keep quiet.
⑪指しゃぶりはやめましょうね	Don't suck your thumb.
⑫よくなるには時間がかかるのよ	It's going to take time to get well.
⑬泣いてもいいよ	It's OK to cry.
⑭いたずらっ子だね	You are a naughty boy.
⑮お昼寝しようね	Take a nap.
⑯童謡を歌おうね	Let's sing a nursery song.
⑰あなたが良くなるためだったら何でもするよ	
	I'll do everything I can to help make you feel better.
⑱絵本はいかが？	Would you like to see a picture book?
⑲プレールームに行きましょうか	Shall we go to the play room?
⑳おやつの時間よ	It's teatime.
㉑もうすぐ夕飯だよ	It's almost time for dinner.
㉒お部屋に帰ろうね	Let's go back to your room.

知っておきたい用語

1）幼児語

ママ	mummy, mommy	パパ	daddy, papa
おばあちゃん	grandma, granny	おじいちゃん	grandpa
おばちゃん	auntie	おじちゃん	uncle
ぽんぽん（腹）	tummy	おへそ	tummy-button, bellybutton
あんよ（foot）	tootsy	おてて（hand）	pud
おしっこ（尿）	pipi（pee）	おしっこをする	take a pee
おねしょ	bed-wetting	大便をする	go poop
わんわん（犬）	bowwow, doggie	にゃんにゃん（猫）	kitty
かえる	froggy		

2）子供の遊び

積み木で遊ぶ	play with blocks	綾取りをする	play cat's cradle
トランプをする	play cards	ビー球遊びをする	play marbles
プラモデルを作る	make model planes	折り紙をする	fold paper
なぞなぞ遊びをする	play riddles	お店ごっこをする	play shop

3）子供の呼称

新生児（生後1ヶ月以内）	neonate
乳児（生後1ヶ月〜1年）	toddler
幼児（生後1年〜3年）	infant
幼児（生後3年〜6年）	preschooler
未熟児	low birth-weight baby

4）子供の病気

水疱瘡	chicken pox
風疹	rubella
はしか	measles
コリック（乳幼児の激しい腹痛）	colic
ジフテリア	diphtheria
ダウン症	Down's syndrome
小児麻痺	poliomyelitis

乳幼児突然死症候群	sudden infant death syndrome, crib death
精神遅滞	mental retardation

5）（親が語る）子供の状態

ひきつけをおこしています	He/She has convulsions.
じんましんが出ています	He/She gets hives.
げっぷが出ます	He/She burps.
おむつかぶれがあります	He/She has diaper rash.
機嫌が悪いです	He/She is irritable.
すごく熱があります	He/She has a high fever.

6）子供入院時の親との会話

坊や（お嬢ちゃん）はどうしましたか	What is the problem with your son（daughter）?
坊や（お嬢ちゃん）ニックネームは何ですか	What is your son's（daughter's）nickname?
坊や（お嬢ちゃん）の好きな食べ物は何ですか	What is your son's（daughter's）favorite food?
毎日病院に来られますか	Can you come to the hospital every day?

解　　答

Exercise 1

1. Visiting hours
2. take a bath
3. lights-out
4. spend the night
5. come back
6. brochure
7. drawer
8. call button
9. valuables
10. pay phone

Exercise 2

1. problem
2. hours　　sleep
3. allergic
4. dizzy
5. diarrhea
6. constipated
7. anemia
8. three times
9. irritated
10. feels heavy

Exercise 3

1. worrying
2. feel free
3. understand
4. afraid
5. worried
6. most worried
7. lonely
8. depression
9. committing suicide
10. talk to

Exercise 4

1. laundry room
2. nurse station
3. rooms
4. dining room
5. patients' lounge
6. emergency exit
7. play room
8. call button
9. smoking area
10. private room

Exercise 5

1. radiotherapy
2. diabetic diet
3. operation
4. shave
5. physical therapy
6. care plan
7. regular diet
8. urinal
9. abdominal breathing
10. rehabilitation

Exercise 6

1. side effects
2. consent form
3. diabetes
4. treatment
5. technical terms
6. therapy
7. pneumonia
8. consent to
9. questions
10. operation

Exercise 7

1. feel the pain
2. mild pain
3. stomachache
4. pain   stop
5. severe pain
6. griping pain
7. painkiller
8. hurts
9. relieve
10. shooting

Exercise 8

1. urine
2. hurt
3. fist
4. pulse   temperature
5. blood pressure
6. 130 over 72
7. thermometer
8. 38.5
9. chest X-rays
10. MRI

Exercise 9

1. wound
2. bandage
3. intravenous injection
4. gauze
5. Stretch   arm
6. Lie on
7. stomach
8. enema
9. hurt
10. shaving

Exercise 10

1. painkiller
2. capsules
3. after each meal
4. antibiotics
5. sleeping pill
6. medicine
7. pills
8. eye drops
9. ointment
10. suppository

Exercise 11

1. over
2. sure   fine
3. give up
4. don't move
5. Shall I
6. take a bath
7. Try to eat
8. smoke
9. let us know
10. lights-out

Exercise 12

1. Congratulations
2. every two months
3. appointment
4. can see
5. pay   cashier
6. come back
7. go home
8. nursing service
9. week
10. for everything

Exercise 13

1. take off
2. clothes   basket
3. laboratory
4. next to
5. draw a map
6. department
7. Go straight
8. Get off the elevator
9. come back
10. pharmacy

Exercise 14

1. surname
2. clinic
3. 239-6742
4. fee 3,000
5. next month
6. 1963
7. fill out
8. restroom
9. detailed examination
10. make an appointment

Glossary　　語彙集

A

a half tablet（1/2錠）69
a pair of crutches（松葉杖）36
a spoonful of（小さじ1杯分の）69
abdominal breathing（腹式呼吸）33, 34, 37
abdominal pain（腹痛）48
acquired immunodeficiency syndrome（後天性免疫不全症候群）42
acute pain（急性の痛み）47
adhesive tape（テープ）64
admission（入院）10
admission window（入院受付）84, 87
after each meal（毎食後）69
after meal（食後に）69
AIDS（エイズ）42
alimentotherapy（食餌療法）35
Alzheimer's disease（アルツハイマー病）42
ampule（アンプル）69
anemia（貧血）15, 16, 41
anesthesia（麻酔）64
anesthesiology（麻酔科）87
anesthetic（麻酔薬）69
aneurysm（脳動脈瘤）42
angina（狭心症）41
anorexia nervosa（神経性食欲不振症）42
antacid medicine（制酸薬）70
antibiotic（抗生物質）68, 69
anticancer drug（抗がん薬）70
antidiabetic（抗糖尿病薬）70
antidiarrhea（止痢剤）70
antidote（解毒剤）70
antifebrile（解熱剤）69
antihistamine（抗ヒスタミン剤）70
antihypertensive agent（降圧薬）69
antiphlogistic（消炎剤）69
antiulcerative（抗潰瘍薬）70
anxiety neurosis（不安神経症）42
anxiety（不安）22, 23
anytime when you have a pain（痛みのあるときに）69
appendicitis（虫垂炎, 盲腸炎）41
appetite（食欲）12, 13
appointed day（予約日）78
armpit（腋の下）54
at the time of rising（起床時）69
arthritis（関節炎）41
artificial feeding（人工栄養）35
artificial respiration（人工呼吸）64
asthma（喘息）41
at bed time（入眠前に）69
as necessary for cough（せきの出るときに）69
as necessary for pain（痛みのあるときに）69
as needed（必要時に）69
athlete's foot（水虫）42
autologous blood transfusion（自己血輸血）25

B

baby food（離乳食）35
backache（腰痛）14
bandage（包帯）63, 64
barium enema examination（直腸バリウム検査）56
Basedow's disease（バセドー氏病）41
bathroom（風呂場）27, 29
be discharged（退院する）10
be hospitalized（入院する）10
be in hospital（入院している）10
bed-pan（便器）36

bedside table（床頭台）35
bedsore（床ずれ）17
bedtime（消灯時間）10
bed-wetting（おねしょ）96
before meal（食前に）69
belches（げっぷ）97
belongings（持ち物）7, 83
between meals（食間に）69
biopsy（生検）57
bite（噛み傷）17
bleary eyes（かすみ眼）15
blister（水疱）17
blocks（積み木）96
blood lab（採血室）88
blood pressure（血圧）33, 52, 54
blood shot of eyes（眼の充血）17
blood test（血液検査）53, 85
blood transfusion（輸血）64
bloody stool（血便）17
bloody urine（血尿）14, 17
bowel movements（便通）13
bowwow（わんわん：犬）96
brain tumor（脳腫瘍）42
breast cancer（乳がん）42
breast feeding（母乳栄養）35
breast milk（母乳）35
brochure（パンフレット）9, 10
bronchitis（気管支炎）41
bruise（打撲傷）17
bump（こぶ）17
burn（やけど）42
burning pain（焼けるような痛み）47

C

Caesarean section（帝王切開）64
cafeteria（食堂）88
call bell（ナースコール）35
call button（ナースコール）8, 9, 28, 35, 60, 66
capsules（カプセル）69, 70
cardiac catheterization（心臓カテーテル検査）56
cardiac diet（心臓病食）35
cardiology（循環器科）87
cardiotonic（強心薬）70
care plan（ケアプラン）32
case worker（ケースワーカー）79
cashier（会計）30, 78, 80, 82, 83, 87
cast（ギプス）64
cat's cradle（綾取り）96
cataract（白内障）42
catheter（カテーテル）64
cell analysis（細胞検査）57
cellular phone（携帯電話）8
chamber-pot（室内トイレ）37
chemotherapy（化学療法）35, 38
chicken pox（水疱瘡）96
chief administrator（事務長）29
Chinese herbal medicine（漢方薬）70
cholagogue（利胆剤）70
chronic pain（慢性の痛み）47
clerk（事務職員）30
clinic（診療所）90
clinical nurse specialist（専門看護師）29
clinical psychologist（臨床心理士）30
close examination（精密検査）91, 92
closet（ロッカー）35
clothing（衣類）35
coin laundry（コインランドリー）11, 29
cold medicine（風邪薬）69
colon cancer（大腸がん）41
colonoscopy（大腸鏡検査）56
coma（昏睡状態）17
commode（カモード）37
compress（湿布）61, 64
computer tomography scan（CTスキャン）56
conjunctivitis（結膜炎）42
consent form（承諾書）39, 40
conservative therapy（内科的治療）35
constipation（便秘）14, 16, 21

consultation room（診察室）27, 88
contagious disease ward（伝染病棟）29
continuous pain（絶え間ない痛み）47
convulsion（ひきつけ）18, 97
coronary care unit（冠状動脈疾患集中治療室）29
corset（コルセット）64
cotton swab（綿棒）64
couch（診察台）83
cough（咳）15, 17
cough medicine（咳止め）69
cramp（けいれん痛）48
cravat（三角巾）64
crust（かさぶた）17
crutch（松葉杖）64
cut（切り傷）17
cutting pain（差し込むような痛み）47
cystitis（膀胱炎）41

D

daily care items（洗面用具）10
deep breath（深呼吸）52
delivery room（分娩室）29
dementia（痴呆）42
dental hygienist（歯科衛生士）30
dental technician（歯科技工士）30
dentistry（歯科）87
dependent（扶養家族）93
depression（うつ状態）23
depression（うつ病）42
dermatology（皮膚科）87
diabetes（糖尿病）40, 41
diabetic diet（糖尿病食）34, 35
dialysis（透析）64
diaper（おむつ）35
diaper rash（おむつかぶれ）97
diarrhea（下痢）14, 16
dietitian（栄養士）30
digestive medicine（消化薬）70
dilation of the pupil（瞳孔散大）17

dining room（食堂）29
diphtheria（ジフテリア）96
discharge（おりもの）19
disinfectant（消毒薬）69
disinfection（消毒）61, 64
dislocation（脱臼）41
diuretic（利尿薬）70
dizzy（めまい）14, 16
doctor（医師）29
doctors' office（医局）29
doggie（わんわん：犬）96
Down's syndrome（ダウン症）96
drawer（引き出し）7, 9
dressing（ガーゼ）64
drugstore（売店）88
dull pain（鈍痛）47

E

eczema（湿疹）17
edema（むくみ）19
electric blanket（電気毛布）35
electrocardiogram（心電図）56
electroencephalogram（脳波）57
electromotive bed（電動ベッド）35
electromyogram（筋電図）57
emergency（緊急時）12
emergency contact（緊急連絡先）93
emergency escape route（避難経路）26
emergency exit（非常口）28, 29, 88
emergency ward（救急病棟）29
endocrinology（内分泌科）87
endoscope（内視鏡）57
endoscopy（内視鏡検査）56
enema（浣腸）61, 63, 64
enema（浣腸器）64
every six hours（6時間ごとに）69
examination couch（診察台）63, 64
eye drops（点眼薬）68, 70
eye patch（眼帯）36
intravenous injection pole（点滴用ポール）36

F

false teeth（入れ歯）35
family doctor（かかりつけ医）81
feel chilly（寒気がする）14
feel shaky（ぞくぞくする）14
feverish（熱っぽい）14
fiberscope（胃ファイバースコープ）57
flash light（懐中電灯）35
florist（花屋）88
taxi stand（タクシー乗り場）88
flu（インフルエンザ）41
fold paper（折り紙をする）96
food poisoning（食中毒）41
fracture（骨折）41
froggy（かえる）96

G

gargle（うがい薬）69
gastric ulcer（胃潰瘍）41
gastritis（胃炎）41
gastrocamera（胃カメラ）57
gastroenterology（消化器科）87
gastroscopy（胃カメラ検査）56
gauze（ガーゼ）63, 64
gene therapy（遺伝子治療）35
general practitioner（一般開業医）81
general reception（総合受付）87
generalized pain（広範囲の痛み）47
glaucoma（緑内障）42
go out（外出する）10
go poop（大便をする）96
gout（痛風）41
granule（顆粒）70
griping pain（きりきりした痛み）46, 47
gruel（粥）35
gynecology（婦人科）87

H

haematinic（造血剤）70
hall（廊下）88
hay fever（花粉症）42
head nurse（病棟師長）29
headache（頭痛）12, 48, 90
health condition（健康状態）12
health insurance（健康保険）20, 81
health insurance card（健康保険証）78, 81, 90, 91, 94
heart attack（心臓発作）41
heart disease（心臓病）41
heart failure（心不全）41
heart murmur（心雑音）17
heartburn（胸焼け）18
heat rash（あせも）42
hemophilia（血友病）41
hepatitis（肝炎）41
hiccup（しゃっくり）14
high fever（高熱）14, 97
hives（じんましん）17, 42, 97
hoarse voice（掠れ声）15
Holter monitor（心電図モニター）57
home-care nursing service（訪問看護サービス）80, 81
hospital director（院長）29
hospital gown（寝衣）7, 35
hospital safe（病院の金庫）10
hospitalization（入院）10
hot water bottle（湯たんぽ）36
hurt（痛む）55
hypertension（高血圧症）41

I

ice pillow（氷枕）36
ID card（診察券）78, 84, 91
immunosuppressant（免疫抑制剤）70
incision（切開）61, 64
incontinent（失禁）14
infant（幼児）96
influenza（インフルエンザ）41
informed consent（インフォームドコンセント）38

inhalant（吸入薬）70
inhalation（吸入）64
inhaler（吸入器）64
injection（注射）61
injector（注射器）64
inpatient（入院患者）10
insomnia（不眠）23, 42
instruction（指示）22
insurance premiums（保険料）81
intensive care unit（集中治療室）29
intermittent pain（断続的な痛み）47
internal medicine（内科）87
international call（国際通話）11
intractable pain（耐えられない痛み）47
intramuscular injection（筋肉注射）64
intravenous drip injection（点滴）60, 61, 64
intravenous injection（静脈注射）63, 64
intubation（挿管）64
irregular pulse（不整脈）56
irritable（機嫌が悪い）97
irritation（いらいら）14
itchy（かゆい）15

J・K
jaundice（黄疸）17
joint pain（関節痛）47
kitty（にゃんにゃん：猫）96

L
lab technician（臨床検査技師）30
laboratory（検査室）85, 88
lack of appetite（食欲不振）23
laundry room（洗濯室）28, 29
laundry service（ランドリーサービス）11
laundry（洗濯物）35
lavatory（トイレ，洗面所）27, 88
laxative（下剤）70
leave the hospital（退院）10, 21, 79, 82
leukemia（白血病）41
licensed practical nurse（准看護師）30

light sensitivity（光過敏）17
lights-out（消灯時間）8-10, 75, 77
liquid diet（流動食）33, 35
liquid（水薬）70
liver cancer（肝臓がん）41
liver cirrhosis（肝硬変）41
liver function test（肝機能検査）57
localized pain（局部的な痛み）47
loose bowel（下痢）14
low birth-weight baby（未熟児）96
low salt diet（減塩食）35
lozenge（咳止めシロップ）69
lumbago（腰痛）47, 48
lump（しこり）17
lung cancer（肺がん）41

M
make model planes（プラモデルを作る）96
manometer（血圧計）57
manual removal of fecal impaction（摘便）64
mealtime（食事時間）10
measles（はしか）41, 96
medical bills（入院費）21
medical social worker（ソーシャルワーカー）30
medicinal therapy（薬物治療）35
medicine（薬）90
memory loss（記憶喪失）18
menopausal disorder（更年期障害）23
mental retardation（精神遅滞）97
midwife（助産師）81
migraine（偏頭痛）18, 48
mild pain（ちょっとした痛み）47
morning sickness（つわり）19
mother's milk（母乳）35
mouthwash（うがい薬）69
mumps（おたふく風邪）41
muscle pain（筋肉痛）48
music therapist（音楽療法士）30
myocardial infarction（心筋梗塞）41

N

nap（お昼寝）95
nationality（国籍）93
nausea（吐き気）14
needle（針）64
neonate（新生児）96
nephritis（腎炎）41
nephrosis（ネフローゼ）41
neurology（神経科）87
neurosurgery（脳神経外科）87
no visitors（面会謝絶）10
nose bleed（鼻血）15
nose drops（点鼻薬）70
numb（しびれ）14
numbness（しびれるような痛み）47
nurse station（ナースステーション）27, 28, 29
nurse's aid（看護助手）30
nursery song（童謡）95
nursery（新生児室）29
nursing department（看護部）29
nutritionist（栄養士）30

O

obstetrics（産科）87
occupation（職業）93
occupational therapist（作業療法士）30
occupational therapy（作業療法）35
ointment（軟膏，塗布薬）68, 70
once a day（1日1回）69
once a day（1日1回）69
one part (unit) measure（1目盛り）69
operation room（手術室）29
operation（手術）18, 32
operator（電話交換手）30
ophthalmology（眼科）87
organ transplantation（臓器移植）35
orthopedics（整形外科）87
orthoptist（視能訓練士）30
osteoporosis（骨粗鬆症）41
otorhinolaryngology（耳鼻咽喉科）87

outpatient department（外来）87
outpatient window（外来窓口）87
over bed table（オーバーベッドテーブル）35
oxygen outlet（酸素プラグ差込口）35

P・Q

painkiller（痛み止め，鎮痛剤）25, 46, 49, 66, 68, 69
pajamas（パジャマ）35
paper diaper（紙オムツ）36
Parkinson's disease（パーキンソン病）42
patients' lounge（談話室）28, 29
pay phone（公衆電話）8, 9, 88
pediatrics（小児科）87
pee（おしっこ）96
perinatal center（周産期センター）29
period（生理）19
persistent pain（しつこい痛み）47
pharmacist（薬剤師）30
pharmacy（薬局）85, 88
physical therapist（理学療法士）30
physical therapy（理学療法）34, 35
physician（医師）29
physiological lab department（生理機能検査室）88
endoscopy department（内視鏡検査室）85, 88
picture book（絵本）95
pill（丸薬）68, 70
pipi（おしっこ）96
plaster（はり薬，湿布薬）70
plastic bandage（ばんそうこう）64
plastic surgery（形成外科）87
play cards（トランプをする）96
play marbles（ビー球遊びをする）96
play shop（お店ごっこをする）96
pneumonia（肺炎）40, 41
poliomyelitis（小児麻痺）96
powder（散剤）70
preschooler（幼児）96
prickling pain（ちくちく痛い）45, 47

primary nurse（プライマリーナース）6
private room（個室）7, 28, 29
prostatic cancer（前立腺癌）41
psychiatry（精神科）87
psychosomatic disorder（心身症）42
psychosomatic medicine（心療内科）85, 87
public health center（保健所）81
public health nurse（保健師）81
public phone（公衆電話）88
pud（おてて）96
pulmonary function test（肺機能検査）56
pulmonology（呼吸器科）87
pus（膿）61, 64
quilt（ふとん）35

R

radiography department（放射線科）88
radiology（放射線科）87
radiotherapy（放射線療法）34, 35, 39
rash（発疹）17
receipt（領収書）78
receptionist（受付係）30
recovery room（回復室）29
rectal cancer（直腸がん）41
referral letter（紹介状）79, 94
referring doctor（紹介医）81
refrigerator（冷蔵庫）35
registered nurse（看護師）30
registration（新患受付）87
regular diet（普通食）33-35
regularly（常用して）13
rehabilitation center（リハビリテーション室）88
rehabilitation（リハビリ）33, 34
religious reason（宗教上の理由）13
resident（研修医）29
respiration rate（呼吸数）56
restroom（トイレ，洗面所）29, 88
rheumatism（リューマチ）41
rigidity（硬直）17

rough skin（肌あれ）19
round（回診）10
rubber air bag（円座）36
rubber sheet（ゴム布）35
rubella（風疹）41, 96
runny nose（鼻水）18

S

scale（体重計）57
scalpel（メス）64
scar（傷あと）17
schizophrenia（精神分裂病）42
scratch（引っかき傷）17
edema（浮腫）17
sedative（鎮静剤）69
sense of fatigue（疲労感）23
serious illness（大きな病気）13
severe pain（ひどい痛み）47
sharp pain（激しい痛み）47
shaving（剃毛）64
shooting pain（うずくような痛み）46, 47
sickroom（病室）29
side effect（副作用）25, 40
sink（洗面台）35
sister（病棟師長）29
skin cancer（皮膚がん）42
sleeping pill（睡眠薬）69
slight fever（微熱）14
slight pain（軽い痛み）47
slippers（上履き）10
smoking area（喫煙所）11, 28, 29
sore throat（のどの痛み）15, 48
speech therapist（言語療法士）30
speech therapy（言語療法）35
spirometer test（肺活量検査）56
spirometer（肺活量計）57
splinter（副木）64
sprain（ねんざ）41
sputum（痰）17
sputum examination（喀痰検査）56

squeezing pain（ぎゅっとくる痛み）47
stabbing pain（ちくちくした痛み）47
staff conference room（会議室）29
stay out（外泊）9, 10
stethoscope（聴診器）57
sting（刺し傷）17
stinging pain（刺すような痛み）47
stomach cancer（胃がん）41
stomach medicine（胃薬）70
stomach ulcer（胃潰瘍）41
stomachache（胃痛）48
stool test（検便）53
stopping the bleeding（止血）64
stretcher（担架）64
stroke（脳卒中）42
student nurse（看護実習生）30
stuffy nose（鼻づまり）18
styptic（止血剤）70
subcutaneous injection（皮下注射）64
sublingual medicine（舌下薬）70
suction（吸引）64
sudden infant death syndrome（乳幼児突然死症候群）97
sundries（日用雑貨）27
superintendent of nurses（看護部長）29
supervisor（管理師長）29
supporter（サポーター）64
suppository（坐薬）68, 70
surgery（外科）87
surgical therapy（外科的治療）35
suture（縫合）64
swelling（腫脹）17
syringe（注射器）64

T

tablet（錠剤）68, 70
take a bath（入浴）7, 9
taking blood sample（採血）53
tea room（喫茶室）88
technical term（専門用語）39, 40
therapy（治療法）38
thermometer（体温計）52, 55, 57
thirty minutes after meal（食後30分後に）69
three times a day（1日3回）69
throbbing pain（ずきずきした痛み）45, 47
thumb-sucking（指しゃぶり）95
tissue cell analysis（細胞検査）57
toddler（乳児）96
toilet（トイレ）88
tongue depressor（舌圧子）64
tonsillitis（扁桃炎）42
toothache（歯痛）18, 48
tootsy（あんよ）96
tourniquet（駆血帯）57
tranquilizer（精神安定剤）69
treatment（治療，処置）40, 42
treatment room（処置室）27, 84, 88
tube feeding（経管栄養）35
tuberculosis（結核）41
tummy（ぽんぽん：おなか）96
tummy-button（おへそ）96
turn off the light（電気を消す）8
tweezers（ピンセット）64
twice a day（1日2回）69
type of insurance（保険証の種類）93

U

ultrasonography（超音波検査法）56
underwear（下着）35
urethral catheterization（導尿）58
urinal（しびん）36
urine test（尿検査）53
urology（泌尿器科）87
uterine cancer（子宮癌）42
uterine myoma（子宮筋腫）42

V

valuables（貴重品）7, 9, 85
vasopressor（昇圧薬）69
visiting hours（面会時間）8, 9

visiting nurse（訪問看護師）81
visitor（面会者，見舞い客）10
vital signs（生命徴候）56
volunteer（ボランティア）30

W

waiting room/area（待合室）87
wake-up time（起床時間）10
walker（歩行器）64
ward（病棟）27, 29
wash basin（洗面器）35
wastebasket（ごみ箱）35
wheel chair（車椅子）36, 64
window（窓口）87
worry（心配ごと）20
wound（傷）63

X

X-ray（X線撮影）56
X-ray department（放射線科）84, 85
X-ray film（X線写真）84
X-ray technician（X線技師）30

監修者・著者紹介

中西睦子（なかにしむつこ）
ミネソタ大学大学院修士課程修了
国際医療福祉大学大学院教授・神戸市看護大学名誉教授

野口ジュディー（のぐち）
神戸学院大学　名誉教授
大阪大学大学院工学研究科　非常勤講師
大阪大学大学院医学系研究科　非常勤講師
神戸大学大学院工学研究科　非常勤講師
神戸大学大学院保健学研究科　非常勤講師

川越栄子（かわごええいこ）
神戸女学院大学大学院文学研究科修士課程修了
神戸女学院大学共通英語教育研究センター教授・センター長
大阪大学・神戸大学医学部非常勤講師

仁平雅子（にへいまさこ）
大阪大学大学院文学研究科博士前期課程修了
元 信州大学医学部附属病院看護師

NDC 490　110p　26cm

耳から学ぶ楽しいナース英語（みみからまなぶたのしいナースえいご）

2002年4月20日　第1刷発行
2024年4月10日　第14刷発行

監修者　中西睦子（なかにしむつこ）
発行者　森田浩章
発行所　株式会社　講談社
　　　　〒112-8001　東京都文京区音羽2-12-21
　　　　販　売　(03)5395-4415
　　　　業　務　(03)5395-3615

KODANSHA

編　集　株式会社　講談社サイエンティフィク
　　　　代表　堀越俊一
　　　　〒162-0825　東京都新宿区神楽坂2-14　ノービィビル
　　　　編　集　(03)3235-3701
印刷所　株式会社双文社印刷・半七写真印刷工業株式会社
製本所　株式会社国宝社

落丁本・乱丁本は，購入書店名を明記のうえ，講談社業務宛にお送り下さい．送料小社負担にてお取替えします．なお，この本の内容についてのお問い合わせは講談社サイエンティフィク宛にお願いいたします．定価はカバーに表示してあります．

© Mutsuko Nakanishi, 2002

本書のコピー，スキャン，デジタル化等の無断複製は著作権法上での例外を除き禁じられています．本書を代行業者等の第三者に依頼してスキャンやデジタル化することはたとえ個人や家庭内の利用でも著作権法違反です．

JCOPY〈(社)出版者著作権管理機構　委託出版物〉
複写される場合は，その都度事前に(社)出版者著作権管理機構（電話 03-3513-6969, FAX 03-3513-6979, e-mail: info@jcopy.or.jp）の許諾を得てください．

Printed in Japan

ISBN4-06-153672-9

講談社の自然科学書

英文ニュースで学ぶ健康とライフスタイル	田中芳文／編著	定価 2,860 円
英語で読む21世紀の健康	阿部祚子・正木美知子／著	定価 1,980 円
大学1年生の なっとく！生物学 第2版	田村隆明／著	定価 2,530 円
大学1年生のなっとく！生態学	鷲谷いづみ／著	定価 2,420 円
亀田講義ナマ中継 有機化学	亀田和久／著	定価 2,420 円
亀田講義ナマ中継 生化学	亀田和久／著	定価 2,530 円
カラー図解 生化学ノート	森 誠／著	定価 2,420 円
ひとりでマスターする生化学	亀井碩哉／著	定価 4,180 円
医学部編入への生命科学演習	松野 彰／監修　井出冬章／著　河合塾KALS／協力	定価 4,730 円
医学部編入への英語演習	河合塾KALS／監修　土田 治／著	定価 4,400 円
好きになる解剖学	竹内修二／著	定価 2,420 円
好きになる解剖学 Part2	竹内修二／著	定価 2,200 円
好きになる解剖学 Part3	竹内修二／著	定価 2,420 円
好きになる解剖学 ミニノート	竹内修二／著	定価 1,760 円
休み時間の免疫学 第3版	齋藤紀先／著	定価 2,200 円
休み時間の解剖生理学	加藤征治／著	定価 2,420 円
Judy先生の英語科学論文の書き方 増補改訂版	野口ジュディーほか／著	定価 3,300 円
できる研究者の論文生産術 どうすれば「たくさん」書けるのか	ポール・J・シルヴィア／著　高橋さきの／訳	定価 1,980 円
PowerPointによる理系学生・研究者のためのビジュアルデザイン入門	田中佐代子／著	定価 2,420 円
新版 理系のためのレポート・論文完全ナビ	見延庄士郎／著	定価 2,090 円
アロマとハーブの薬理学	川口健夫／著	定価 2,640 円
学振申請書の書き方とコツ 改訂第2版	大上雅史／著	定価 2,750 円
できる研究者の論文作成メソッド 書き上げるための実践ポイント	ポール・J・シルヴィア／著　高橋さきの／訳	定価 2,200 円

※表示価格には消費税（10%）が加算されています。　「2024年4月現在」

講談社サイエンティフィク　https://www.kspub.co.jp/